White Talking Therapy Can't Think in Black!

A Journey Through Systemic Biases to Inclusivity and Mental Health Empowerment.

By

Jarell Bempong

© Jarell Bempong 2023

Terms and Conditions

LEGAL NOTICE

© Copyright 2023 ©**jarellbempong**

All rights reserved. The content contained within this book may not be reproduced, duplicated, or transmitted without direct written permission from the author or the publisher. Email requests to kevin@babystepspublishing.com

Under no circumstances will any blame or legal responsibility be held against the publisher, or author for any damages, reparation, or monetary loss due to the information contained within this book, either directly or indirectly.

Legal Notice:

This book is copyright protected. It is only for personal use. You cannot amend, distribute, sell, use, quote, or paraphrase any part of the content within this book without the author's or publisher's consent.

Disclaimer Notice:

Please note that the information contained within this document is for educational and entertainment purposes only. All effort has been executed to present accurate, up-to-date, reliable, and complete information. No warranties of any kind are declared or implied. Readers acknowledge that the author is not engaging in the rendering of legal, financial, medical, or professional advice. The content within this book has been derived from various sources. Please consult a licensed professional before attempting any techniques outlined in this book.

By reading this document, the reader agrees that under no circumstances is the author responsible for any direct or indirect losses incurred due to the use of the information contained within this document, including, but not limited to, errors, omissions, or inaccuracies.

Published by Babysteps Publishing Limited, All enquires to kevin@babystepspublishing.com

ISBN- 9798854813570

Table of Contents

Notice From The Author   1

Why I Wrote This Book   5

Who Did I Write This Book For?   7

Chapter 1: Systemic Racism in Mental Health Care: Unveiling the Historical Roots   17

Chapter 2: Unpacking Biases and Fostering Cultural Consciousness: Empowering Individuals   49

Chapter 3: Culturally Conscious Care: 77

Chapter 4: Antiracism and Allyship: 115

Chapter 5: Creating Inclusive Workplaces: 149

Chapter 6: Dismantling Racism, Promoting Mental Health: Empowering Individuals for Change   183

About the Author   225

Services by Jarell Bempong: Expanding the Journey   229

Notice From The Author

I acknowledge that the terms "Black people" and "people of colour" or "people of African" descent encompass a wide range of racial and ethnic identities, and I recognise the diverse experiences of Black individuals and other cultural minorities. This book's core is a call to action for allyship, anti-racism, anti-homophobia, and other forms of discrimination. I have strived to be respectful and inclusive in my writing. Still, I acknowledge that my experiences as a Black person reflect the systemic racism, discrimination, and various forms of oppression faced by Black individuals and other cultural minority communities. In my book, "White Talking Therapy Can't Think in Black! - A Journey Through Systemic Biases to Inclusivity and Mental Health Empowerment," I use these terms to refer to individuals who have historically experienced oppression and marginalisation within Western society, including Black individuals and other cultural minorities.

When I speak of "White People," I am also mindful that White people encompass many racial and ethnic identities. While I strive to be respectful and inclusive when talking about White people, I also acknowledge the privilege afforded them by a systemically racist society. I also recognise that White people may have experienced discrimination and marginalisation but do not undergo the same systemic racism and bigotry as Black people and other cultural minorities. Challenging and dismantling the power dynamics embedded in our society is crucial.

This book promotes inclusivity, understanding, and empathy for all individuals. It aims to shed light on the historical and ongoing disparities in mental health care, specifically focusing on the experiences of marginalised communities. By highlighting these issues, I call upon readers, regardless of their racial or ethnic background, to actively engage in allyship and anti-racist practices. This includes challenging systems of oppression and discrimination, including homophobia and other forms of bigotry, to create a more equitable and inclusive mental health care system.

While acknowledging different communities' unique experiences and perspectives, I aim to address the common thread of oppression that ties marginalised communities together. By doing so, we can work towards dismantling systemic barriers and promoting inclusivity in mental health care for all individuals. This book is not about singling out any particular group of people but examining the pervasive impact of racism and inequality on the development of contemporary psychology.

This book is not just an academic exercise but a call to action. It urges all of us to stand up and fight for the rights and dignity of every individual, regardless of race, gender, or any other identifier. Let us actively challenge and dismantle systems of oppression and discrimination. By fostering allyship, anti-racism, anti-homophobia, and other forms of discrimination, we can create a world where mental health is a fundamental human right, not a privilege.

I invite you to join me in exploring how racism, homophobia, and other forms of discrimination shape our lives and world. It may be challenging and uncomfortable, but it is necessary for progress towards a brighter and more equitable future. Although the path ahead may be difficult, I am confident that together, we can create a world where mental health is prioritised, and everyone is valued and treated with the respect they deserve. Let us embark on this journey together and not rest until we have achieved true equality and inclusivity.

Why I Wrote This Book

I wrote this book, "White Talking Therapy Can't Think in Black! - A Journey Through Systemic Biases to Inclusivity and Mental Health Empowerment," to address the pervasive discrimination within the mental health care system, the workplace, and society. Drawing from personal and professional experiences, I witnessed firsthand the detrimental effects of a whitewashed mental health curriculum and the alarming prevalence of discrimination in mental health care settings.

In this groundbreaking book, "Culturally Responsive Mental Health Care: Empowering Professionals, Transforming the Workplace, and Beyond," I serve as a whistle-blower, exposing the hidden truths and injustices of systemic racism within the mental health care system. By sharing personal and professional experiences, I shed light on the disparities and biases in therapy, workplaces, and society, urging readers to examine and challenge these ingrained structures critically.

I delve into the complexities of antiracism, allyship, cultural consciousness, and effective communication, equipping mental health professionals with the necessary tools to create inclusively and empowering therapeutic environments. Furthermore, I expand the scope beyond therapy, exploring how these principles can be applied to the broader workplace and society. I believe that dismantling systemic racism and fostering cultural consciousness is essential for the well-being and success of individuals in all facets of life.

In this book, I offer insights and strategies for mental health professionals seeking to navigate the challenges of providing culturally responsive care. I guide people in recognising and addressing personal biases, actively engaging in antiracist practises, and fostering allyship with marginalised communities. By challenging the status quo and embracing cultural consciousness, mental health professionals can play a pivotal role in transforming the mental health care system and promoting equity and inclusivity.

Additionally, I extend the discussion to the workplace, recognising that systemic racism and discrimination affect individuals beyond therapy sessions. I explore how organisations and leaders can cultivate inclusive work environments that prioritise the mental well-being of all employees. By examining the intersectionality of race, culture, and mental health in the workplace, I provide practical strategies to foster an inclusive culture, promote diversity, and address racial disparities.

This book aims to empower mental health professionals, the workforce, and individuals to actively contribute to a society free from systemic racism and discrimination. By amplifying the voices of marginalised communities, challenging ingrained biases, and promoting cultural consciousness, we can collectively create a mental health care system, workplaces, and a society that values and supports the well-being of all individuals, regardless of their racial or cultural background.

Who Did I Write This Book For?

I wrote this book, "White Talking Therapy Can't Think in Black! - A Journey Through Systemic Biases to Inclusivity and Mental Health Empowerment," primarily focusing on individuals seeking empowerment and understanding in navigating the mental health care system, workplace dynamics, and societal structures.

For individuals, I aim to provide insights and tools to help them recognise and challenge the impact of systemic racism on their mental health and well-being. This book offers validation and support for those who have experienced discrimination within the mental health care system or the workplace. It equips individuals with strategies to advocate for themselves, navigate oppressive systems, and seek culturally responsive care. By sharing personal and professional experiences, I hope to foster a sense of empowerment and provide a resource for personal growth and healing.

Furthermore, I wrote this book with mental health professionals in mind, recognising their crucial role in providing effective and inclusive care. By sharing insights, research, and practical strategies, I aim to equip mental health professionals with the knowledge and tools to address systemic racism within their practice. This book guides professionals in recognising and addressing personal biases, fostering cultural consciousness, and creating therapeutic environments that embrace diversity and promote the well-being of all clients. By amplifying the voices of marginalised communities and promoting antiracist practices, mental health professionals can contribute to transforming the mental health care system and fostering a more equitable society.

Additionally, I extend the discussion to the workplace, recognising that systemic racism and discrimination impact individuals beyond therapy sessions. This book addresses the intersectionality of race, culture, and mental health in work environments, providing insights and strategies for employers, human resources professionals, and organisational leaders. It explores how organisations can cultivate inclusive and supportive work environments that prioritise the mental well-being of all employees. By examining biases, promoting diversity, and addressing racial disparities in the workplace, this book aims to inspire positive change and create equitable and empowering workplaces.

In summary, "Decolonising Mental Health" is written for individuals seeking empowerment, mental health professionals aiming to provide inclusive care, and workplaces striving to create supportive and equitable environments. It serves as a resource that empowers individuals to navigate discriminatory systems, challenges biases and fosters cultural consciousness. For mental health professionals and workplaces, it provides insights and strategies to promote inclusivity, address systemic racism, and prioritise the mental well-being of all individuals.

Ananse's and the Golden Key: A Tale of Freedom and Self-Rediscovery

Deep within the lush African forest, where the foliage whispered secrets and sunlight danced through the leaves, Ananse the Spider was an expert weaver of intricate webs. Every day, he delighted in the symphony of nature, blissfully unaware of the impending darkness that loomed overhead. One fateful day, a solemn breeze carried whispers of despair to Ananse's sensitive ears, piercing his heart like an arrow. The black spiders of the forest, his brethren, were trapped in the clutches of mental enslavement by a nefarious white owl known as the White Owl of Suppression. Ananse knew he must embark on a perilous journey to liberate their minds and restore their identities.

With unwavering determination, Ananse set forth, his eight legs carrying him swiftly through the verdant wilderness. The forest path presented a labyrinth of ancient trees, their gnarled branches stretching like skeletal arms towards the heavens. A symphony of calls and rustling leaves accompanied his every step, reminding him of the delicate balance of nature.

As he traversed the treacherous terrain, Ananse encountered several peculiar characters who tested his wit and cunning. The first was a majestic elephant, wise and venerable, who shared tales of forgotten wisdom. Ananse cautiously approached the great creature, seeking guidance on liberating his brethren from the White Owl's grasp. The elephant's eyes, reflecting understanding beyond time, offered a cryptic riddle that promised a hint of truth. Ananse, ever the trickster, deciphered the riddle's enigmatic meaning with elegant precision, realising that the elephant's knowledge only scratched the surface of liberation.

Continuing his journey, Ananse stumbled upon mischievous woodland sprites, their laughter echoing. Drawn to their infectious merriment, they proposed an alliance, pledging their aid in exchange for a share of the forest's hidden treasures. Ananse's instincts, honed by generations of spider cunning, alerted him to their deceptive nature. He spun a web of words, skilfully deceiving the sprites into abandoning their greedy intentions. Alone once more, Ananse pressed onward, knowing the fate of his brethren rested upon his silk-strung shoulders.

Finally, Ananse encountered Asaase Yaa, the ethereal goddess of the earth, radiating an aura of tranquillity. She possessed a profound understanding of the pain that gripped the hearts of the black spiders. Compassionately moved by their plight, Asaase Yaa bestowed upon Ananse a golden key, its surface shimmering with ancient symbols. This key, she explained, held the power of cultural consciousness—a tangible manifestation of liberation and self-discovery.

Grateful for the goddess's benevolence, Ananse bowed deeply, his limbs trembling with reverence and determination. Clutching the golden key close to his thorax, he felt its weight as both a responsibility and an emblem of hope. Renewed by his encounter with Asaase Yaa, Ananse ventured deeper into the forest, the path before him shrouded in both shadow and possibility.

Finally, Ananse arrived at the forest's heart, where the air grew thick with tension. There, perched on a lofty branch, was the White Owl of Suppression, his pure feathers starkly contrasting against the night sky. The owl's piercing gaze bore into Ananse, an unsettling mixture of arrogance and malice. Undeterred, Ananse summoned his courage, knowing the time for action had come.

With the golden key clutched tightly, Ananse approached the White Owl, his voice resolute and unwavering. As the owl's laughter reverberated through the canopy, a chorus of tiny arachnid hearts pounded in anticipation. Ananse inserted the key into the ethereal lock, and with a resounding click, the mental shackles that bound his brethren shattered like fragile glass.

Once held captive by the White Owl's nefarious enchantment, the black spiders felt a surge of liberation wash over their beings. Their eight legs quivered with newfound strength, and their minds blossomed with vibrant hues of individuality. The White Owl, eyes wide with disbelief, attempted to reassert his control, but the winds of change had already swept through the forest, carrying away his dominion.

In a triumph of wisdom and resilience, Ananse emerged victorious, freeing his brethren from the clutches of the White Owl's suppression. Gratitude swelled within the hearts of the black spiders, who bestowed upon Ananse the title of Guardian of Identity. The forest abounded with jubilant celebrations as newfound freedom weaved a tapestry of unity among the inhabitants.

And so, the tale of Ananse and the golden key resonated throughout the annals of time, a timeless reminder of the power of self-discovery and the enduring importance of cultural identity. Generations to come would recount the tale, their voices filled with awe and inspiration, as they learned to navigate the labyrinth of life with wit, courage, and an unwavering belief in the transformative power of freedom.

Unleashing Cultural Consciousness: Ananse's Journey to Mental Liberation

In cultural psychology, the story of Ananse and the key to cultural consciousness is a testament to the profound impact that black culture can have on modern psychology. This captivating tale embodies the essence of cultural consciousness therapy and African therapy. It is a powerful tool for individuals to explore their cultural identity and restore their mental well-being.

Ananse, the clever spider at the story's heart, represents the reservoir of African wisdom and resilience. As he embarks on his heroic journey, encountering obstacles and adversaries, he becomes an allegory for the struggles. Black individuals face a world often plagued by whitewashing and discrimination. Through his triumphs, Ananse displays the strength and ingenuity that lie within cultural heritage.

Using African stories like Ananse's within therapeutic sessions allows Black individuals to reconnect with their cultural roots. These narratives provide a unique lens through which individuals can explore their identity, finding solace, inspiration, and empowerment. Individuals can reclaim narratives that have been overshadowed or misrepresented by delving into these tales, thereby dismantling the chains of mental enslavement.

Ananse's encounters with the wise owl and mischievous monkeys mirror the complexities and challenges of mental health. The story underscores the importance of seeking solutions through a cultural lens, recognising that mainstream approaches may only partially address marginalised communities' unique experiences and perspectives. Ananse's ability to outsmart these characters signifies the power of cultural wisdom in navigating mental health challenges and finding paths to liberation.

Crucially, the story also emphasises the significance of community and collective healing. Ananse's unwavering determination to free his fellow spiders from mental enslavement stems from his compassion and responsibility towards his community. The ultimate liberation of the black spiders, achieved through collective effort, highlights the transformative potential of unity and support in the face of adversity.

Incorporating stories like Ananse's into therapy sessions provide individuals with inspiration and resilience rooted in their cultural heritage. By embracing their cultural consciousness, individuals can draw strength from the wisdom of their ancestors and confront the multifaceted challenges of mental health with increased confidence and fortitude. Moreover, cultural consciousness therapy and African therapy empower individuals to face systemic oppression and discrimination head-on, fostering the reclamation of their identities and nurturing a profound sense of self-worth.

The story of Ananse and the key to cultural consciousness weave together the intricate tapestry of Black culture, psychology, and healing. It serves as a potent reminder that by honouring and integrating cultural identity within therapeutic frameworks, individuals can embark on a transformative journey towards self-discovery, growth, and holistic well-being.

"Guided by empathy, we confront racism's hidden scars in mental health care. Together, we create a future of inclusivity and well-being, both in the workplace and society."

- Jarell Bempong

Chapter 1

Systemic Racism in Mental Health Care: Unveiling the Historical Roots

Imagine, an intricate tapestry representing the interconnected domains of mental health care, workplaces, and society. The design is vast and colourful, woven from the diverse threads of human experiences. This tapestry appears harmonious, symbolising the potential for healing, growth, and a flourishing life.

Yet, a closer examination reveals the flaws hidden within. Although standing as a stronghold built on empathy and understanding, the mental health care system conceals within its walls a complexity of inequality. Systemic racism and white supremacy have been woven into its structure, casting dark shadows over those seeking refuge.

The workplace, too, unfolds as a lively part of this fabric, rich with diverse talents and ambitions. It should be a space where everyone, irrespective of race, can weave their dreams into reality. But the threads of systemic racism are also entwined here, distorting its true essence and holding back individuals from reaching their fullest potential.

Extend your gaze to society, and you will find that the marks of systemic racism stretch beyond individual institutions. They reach into the very weave of our communities, creating uneven textures and barriers that hinder the journey towards equality. They manifest in the fabric of our social norms, biases, and practices that unevenly distribute opportunities, casting a shadow over our collective well-being.

This chapter will carefully unpick these tangled threads to understand how white supremacy and systemic racism have subtly woven into our everyday lives. With a keen eye and a commitment to change, we will work to mend this tapestry, striving for a future where mental health care, the workplace, and society become emblematic of inclusivity, equity, and shared prosperity. By addressing the imperfections in our communal fabric, we can create a tapestry that genuinely reflects the beauty and potential within us all.

A Comprehensive Examination of White Supremacist Ideology: Historical Roots and Modern Manifestations

White supremacist thinking, a belief system centred around the inherent superiority of the white race over other racial and ethnic groups, has a profoundly intricate and disturbing history. This ideology has shaped the modern world and continues to resonate within our societies. To comprehensively understand its genesis and evolution, we must scrutinise its historical origins, influential figures, terminology, and varying manifestations across different epochs.

The Emergence of White Supremacy

The seeds of white supremacist ideology were sown during the era of European colonialism and the transatlantic slave trade, which commenced in the 15th century. The expansionist European powers required a justification for their imperial conquests and the ensuing subjugation of indigenous peoples. They found this in the conception of racial superiority, suggesting that some races, particularly those of European descent, were inherently more advanced, civilised, and deserving of rulership over others.

Scientific Racism and Pseudoscientific Theories

During the 18th and 19th centuries, this insidious belief system began to wear the mask of science, leading to the emergence of scientific racism. Under this guise, pseudoscientific theories flourished, such as Social Darwinism and phrenology.

After Charles Darwin's influential "On the Origin of Species" (1859), Social Darwinism misappropriated Darwin's theory of natural selection, extending it to human races. The idea of survival of the fittest was contorted to propose that the white race, deemed the most advanced, was destined to dominate others.

Simultaneously, phrenology surfaced, claiming that character and intelligence were products of an individual's skull shape and size. This false premise buttressed racial stereotypes, asserting certain races' inherent intelligence or moral superiority based on cranial measurements.

Extreme Manifestations of White Supremacist Ideology: The Ku Klux Klan and Eugenics

In the United States, white supremacist ideology manifested in a particularly malevolent form with the emergence of the Ku Klux Klan (KKK) in 1865, post the Civil War. The KKK and other white supremacist groups employed terror and violence to suppress African Americans and other minority groups, thus striving to uphold white dominance and prevent social and political equality.

The 20th century witnessed the rise of eugenics, a pseudo-scientific movement advocating selective breeding to ostensibly improve the genetic quality of the human population. Proponents of eugenics often backed white supremacist ideas, promoting policies that sought to prevent the reproduction of individuals considered "unfit" or racially inferior.

The Holocaust and the Unspoken African Victims

The Holocaust during World War II remains one of the most horrifying manifestations of white supremacist thinking. Adolf Hitler's Nazi regime implemented a genocidal program to exterminate millions of Jews, Romani people, people with disabilities, homosexuals, and other minority groups due to their perceived racial and social inferiority. Among the myriad victims of this tragedy were also African and Afro-German individuals, whose stories are often eclipsed in mainstream Holocaust narratives.

While there is a lack of comprehensive documentation, historians estimate that thousands of African and Afro-German individuals were subjected to sterilisation, medical experimentation, detention, and murder during the Nazi regime. These individuals were targeted under racially motivated eugenics policies and pseudoscientific theories that formed the backbone of Hitler's Aryan supremacy ideology. This often-overlooked aspect of the Holocaust further underscores the wide-reaching and catastrophic consequences of white supremacist ideology when taken to its extreme.

King Leopold II of Belgium: Colonial Atrocities in the Congo

Another manifestation of white supremacy with devastating human consequences can be seen in the brutal colonial rule of King Leopold II of Belgium over the Congo Free State (now the Democratic Republic of Congo) from 1885 to 1908. This period is infamously known for its severe exploitation and human rights abuses of the indigenous population.

Lured by the prospects of ivory and rubber, which were in high demand in the global market, Leopold II implemented a reign of terror, using forced labour, systematic brutality, and violence to extract these valuable resources. He established a regime so brutal and exploitative that it significantly reduced the Congolese population, with estimated deaths ranging from several million to 10 million indigenous people.

The atrocities committed by Leopold II, mainly under the guise of "civilising" the African population, provide a chilling example of white supremacist ideology put into practice. These instances of colonial violence and genocide highlight the dire need for historical education and recognition of these atrocities to combat the enduring influence of white supremacy.

White Supremacy in the Modern World

Despite significant progress made by the mid-20th century civil rights movement in dismantling overt white supremacist practices, the ideology has persisted, often in more insidious ways. Modern-day white supremacy frequently operates covertly, fueled by hate speech, online radicalisation, and racist rhetoric. The rise of far-right movements and white nationalist groups, such as the alt-right and Identitarian movements, signify a concerning trend that emphasises the enduring influence of white supremacist thinking.

The African Connection: How European Colonisation Shaped Modern Psychology and the Urgent Need for Inclusive Mental Health Care

As a field of study, psychology has evolved and developed over time, reflecting the dominant perspectives and ideologies of the societies in which it emerged. Unfortunately, the history of psychology is deeply intertwined with the concept of White supremacy and its resulting racism, which has had a lasting impact on the field and its approach to mental health care. Despite the abolition of slavery and growing awareness of the devastating effects of slavery, colonialism, and neo-colonialism on Africa and her diaspora countries, communities of colour have been excluded from the discourse of mental health care, perpetuating inequalities and limiting access to culturally conscious support. This chapter aims to delve deeper into the connections between White supremacy, racism, and modern psychology, shedding light on the historical injustices that continue to shape mental health care today.

This chapter will carefully unpick these tangled threads to understand how white supremacy and systemic racism have subtly woven into our everyday lives. With a keen eye and a commitment to change, we will work to mend this tapestry, striving for a future where mental health care, the workplace, and society become emblematic of inclusivity, equity, and shared prosperity. By addressing the imperfections in our communal fabric, we can create a tapestry that genuinely reflects the beauty and potential within us all.

Decoding Racism's Legacy in Psychotherapy: A Journey from Colonial Shadows to Culturally Conscious Healing

As we traverse the intricate labyrinth of our shared history, it is impossible to ignore colonialism's profound, lingering shadow on societies worldwide. The roots of this legacy are woven with stigma, disregard, and limited resources, all residues of white supremacist ideologies that fuelled the "White Man's Burden" - the disquieting concept employed to justify the conquest and subjugation of indigenous peoples by European powers during the era of colonialism and the transatlantic slave trade. This section continues the narrative by examining white supremacist ideologies, unravelling their enduring effects on diverse communities and regions, particularly the birth and development of modern psychotherapy.

Phase I: Slavery and Colonisation: A Prelude to Systemic Oppression (15th to 19th Centuries)

1.1 Slavery: The Genesis of Systemic Oppression

The Portuguese ushered in a devastating chapter in human history in 1441 with the initiation of the transatlantic slave trade. This inhuman institution of chattel slavery, especially in the Americas, subjected African people to unspeakable trauma and laid the groundwork for the ongoing oppression of Black individuals.

1.2 Colonisation: Deepening Racial Hierarchies

In 1492, the tide of colonisation rolled in with European powers' incursions into the Americas. This invasion triggered the setup of plantation systems, exploiting indigenous populations and leading to the displacement and subjugation of native peoples. This process bolstered existing racial hierarchies and fortified systems of racial discrimination.

1.3 English Involvement and the Expansion of the Slave Trade

From 1555 onwards, English involvement in the slave trade deepened, punctuated by critical milestones such as establishing The Company of Adventurers of London Trading into the Parts of Africa in 1618 and The Royal African Company's formation in 1672. With the disbandment of the Royal African Company's monopoly in 1698, the trade routes opened to private traders from Bristol and Liverpool, further entrenching the destructive system.

Phase II: The Emergence of Modern Psychotherapy: Echoing Eurocentric Perspectives (Late 19th to Early 20th Century)

2.1 Foundational Psychology: Eurocentric Origins

The roots of modern psychotherapy took hold in the late 19th century, guided by key figures such as Wilhelm Wundt, Sigmund Freud, and William James. However, these trailblazers' theories bore the unmistakable imprint of Eurocentric perspectives, tainted by the prevailing racial biases of their era.

2.2 The Advent of Clinical Psychology and Intelligence Testing

Thanks to pioneers like Lightner Witmer and Alfred Binet, significant developments in clinical psychology and intelligence testing extended the reach of psychological studies. However, these advances remained steeped in Eurocentric perspectives, ignoring the unique experiences of non-European populations.

2.3 Paradigm Shifts: Behaviorism and Humanistic Psychology

The rise of behaviourism, pioneered by John B. Watson, and humanistic psychology, spearheaded by Carl Rogers and Abraham Maslow, marked essential psychological shifts. Nevertheless, the spectre of Eurocentric dominance still loomed large.

Phase III: Pathologising Blackness: The Echoes of Scientific Racism

The emergence of scientific racism during the 18th and 19th centuries gave impetus to the narrative of racial hierarchy, further devaluing the stature of Black individuals. These flawed theories, falsely garbed in the guise of scientific fact, justified the enslavement and subjugation of Africans, thereby shaping societal beliefs and attitudes towards mental health.

Phase IV: The Limitations of Early Psychotherapy: Eurocentrism and its Impact on Marginalised Communities

Freud's theories, influenced by the racial biases of his time, contributed to the pathologisation of Blackness. His theories overlooked cultural context, embedding a Eurocentric lens in therapeutic frameworks and marginalising Black communities' experiences and healing practices.

Phase V: The Persistence of Eurocentric Dominance in Psychotherapy

Eurocentric dominance continued its stronghold throughout the late 19th and early 20th centuries, overshadowing contributions from non-European cultures. The impact of this Eurocentric slant in psychotherapy marginalised these cultures, failing to acknowledge their unique cultural practices and healing traditions.

Phase VI: The Imprint of Eurocentric Psychotherapy on Non-European Cultures: Decoding Marginalisation and the Quest for Cultural Consciousness

The colonial expansion of Western powers resulted in the imposition of Western perspectives upon colonised peoples. Indigenous healing traditions and non-white perspectives were pushed to the margins and dismissed by Eurocentric models, leading to a systemic imbalance in psychotherapy.

Phase VII: The Continuation of Power Imbalances: From Slavery to Neocolonialism

From the era of slavery to the advent of neocolonialism, power imbalances were preserved and mirrored in the development and practice of psychotherapy. Unless these imbalances are actively dismantled, psychotherapy risks reinforcing racial disparities and perpetuating the marginalisation of individuals from diverse cultural backgrounds.

Towards a Culturally Conscious Psychotherapy

The interconnected histories of slavery, colonisation, and modern psychotherapy underscore the enduring influence on mental health. To pave the way for an inclusive mental health landscape, we must acknowledge historical misdeeds, dismantle racist roots, and challenge Eurocentric biases.

The Birth of Modern Psychotherapy: A Dark Historical Link

What if the roots of psychotherapy were entangled with humanity's darkest aspects? This part explores the uncomfortable truths about psychotherapy's origins and the haunting legacy of racism. This section explores significant figures and events that shaped psychotherapy, from social evolution theories to medicalising slavery. It also exposes connections between prominent psychologists and colonial activities, revealing a deeply ingrained racial bias.

As we embark on a quest through the winding corridors of time, prepare to unearth instances that vividly expose the disconcerting intersection of mental health practices and systemic bigotry. Brace yourself for a voyage that might stir discomfort but is indispensable in our pursuit of justice and enlightenment.

The horrifying examples of racially influenced diagnoses include:

Drapetomania: This term coined by American physician Samuel A. Cartwright in the 19th century labelled the urge of enslaved people to escape from their captors as a mental disorder. Cartwright's erroneous assertion of innate racial inferiority falsely pathologised the human yearning for freedom.

Neurasthenia: Employed frequently during the late 19th and early 20th centuries, this diagnosis sought to explain cultural and racial differences, pathologising individuals from colonised or minority communities as deficient in the vitality and motivation typically associated with white, Western individuals.

Hysteria: This diagnosis was a tool to pathologise and stereotype women, especially women of colour, portraying them as emotionally unstable and incapable of logical thought or behaviour.

Cultural Insanity: This term stigmatised individuals perceived to suffer mental illness due to their cultural background or beliefs. It worked to pathologise Indigenous or minority cultures, rationalising the supposed "civilising mission" of colonialism.

Hyperemotionality: This label was attributed to individuals from colonised or minority communities deemed overly emotional and lacking the calm demeanour of white, Western individuals.

Atavistic Insanity: This diagnosis stigmatised individuals from colonised or minority communities, associating their mental illnesses with supposed primitive traits they possessed.

Ethnopsychiatry: Although the term initially referred to the study of mental health and illness in diverse cultures and ethnic groups, it was frequently used derogatorily to stereotype and pathologise non-Western cultures and lifestyles.

Pathological Nostalgia: This term pathologised the homesickness experienced by enslaved individuals uprooted from their native lands and transported to the Americas as part of the transatlantic slave trade.

The outlined diagnoses and concepts nurtured harmful stereotypes and prejudices and justified exploitative and oppressive practices. Although contemporary mental health professionals have denounced these diagnoses, their historical usage underscores the necessity for continuous critical scrutiny of biases and prejudices in mental health. It emphasises the need for culturally conscious care for all individuals.

Shining a Light on the Dark Corners of Psychology: Racial Bias in the Ideologies of Early Pioneers

To understand the enduring footprint of colonial ideologies on psychology, we must unflinchingly delve into the discriminatory and harmful racial beliefs harboured by its early pioneers. This crucial exploration elucidates the colonial ideologies' effects on the evolution of psychology and the consequent systemic bias. Moreover, it illuminates the ongoing struggle to dismantle these biases and establish more inclusive practices in mental healthcare.

Sigmund Freud: As a monumental figure in psychology, Freud's theories endorsed stereotypes and propagated essentialist views of race. He argued that certain races were innately inferior, basing these claims on biological and genetic determinants. His theories were also marked by sexism, perceiving women as inherently subordinate to men.

Carl Jung: Jung, another luminary in the field, approached psychology with a distinctly Eurocentric lens, perpetuating stereotypes about non-European cultures. He depicted these societies as rudimentary and intellectually underdeveloped compared to Western civilisations, solidifying the power dynamic between colonisers and the colonised.

Henri Stern: Stern, a prominent French psychologist, adhered to a hierarchical view of race, suggesting the inherent superiority or inferiority of certain races. His beliefs contributed to the derogation and marginalisation of non-European communities by depicting them as intellectually undeveloped and primitive.

William McDougall: McDougall, a British psychologist, advocated a racial hierarchy, asserting that innate characteristics determined the superiority or inferiority of certain races. Such beliefs helped cement systemic bias within psychology.

Francis Galton: Galton, the founder of eugenics, advanced theories promoting the enhancement of the human race via selective breeding. He propagated the notion of a racial hierarchy, with white Europeans perceived as superior to other racial groups. His ideas profoundly influenced psychology and subsequent social policies and practices.

Richard von Krafft-Ebing: An Austrian psychiatrist, Krafft-Ebing is renowned for his work on psychopathology and sexual disorders. However, his theories on racial degeneration and the pathologisation of non-European races reflect entrenched racist ideologies. His writings fostered the notion that certain races were predisposed to mental illness and moral decay, reinforcing harmful stereotypes and stigmatisation.

Alfred Binet: Known for developing the first modern intelligence test, Binet's research wasn't free from racial biases. He endorsed racial hierarchies and proposed that genetic factors influenced intelligence, implying inherent intellectual inferiority in specific racial backgrounds. Binet's work entrenched systemic discrimination in intelligence testing and fortified discriminatory practices.

Lewis Terman: An American psychologist renowned for his work in intelligence testing and contribution to the Stanford-Binet Intelligence Scales, Terman's research had a robust racist underpinning. He utilised I.Q. tests to justify racial segregation and immigration restrictions, fostering harmful stereotypes and discriminatory practices.

Carl Brigham: Brigham, another American psychologist, contributed significantly to developing standardised intelligence tests, including the SAT. He harboured profound racial biases and authored "A Study of American Intelligence," claiming white Americans' innate intellectual superiority over immigrants and people of colour. His work fortified racial stereotypes and provided a pseudo-scientific foundation for discriminatory policies.

John Watson: Watson, a prominent American psychologist and behaviourism founder, held racist views mirroring his era's prevailing attitudes. He endorsed eugenics, arguing for the white race's superiority. His theories focus solely on observable behaviour, marginalised non-white communities, and neglect systemic racism's impact on mental health.

Gustave Le Bon: Le Bon, a French social psychologist, theorised about racial and cultural superiority. He contended that Western civilisation was inherently superior to non-European cultures, whom he viewed as less evolved and prone to irrational behaviour. His theories contributed to the persistence of racial stereotypes and the marginalisation of non-Western viewpoints.

By probing psychology's ideological and historical underpinnings, we can discern the origins of racism and discrimination in mental healthcare. This knowledge urges us to confront these biases, foster cultural consciousness, and strive for a more equitable mental healthcare approach that honours and respects all individuals' diverse identities and experiences.

The Echo of Early Ideologies in Modern Psychology:

The ideologies of early pioneers like Freud, Jung, and Galton have left enduring footprints on psychology, even in contemporary practice. The Eurocentric bias, gender discrimination, and racial prejudice in their theories continue to influence diagnostic criteria, clinical assessments, and mental health treatment approaches.

1. **Eurocentric Bias in Diagnostic Criteria:** The diagnostic criteria often fail to capture individuals' unique mental health experiences from diverse racial and cultural backgrounds. This is an ongoing reflection of the Eurocentric perspectives promoted by early pioneers.

2. **Gender Discrimination:** The sexism inherent in some early theories has shaped stereotypes that continue to affect how women's mental health is perceived and treated today.

3. **Racial Prejudice in Clinical Assessments:** Assessment biases can lead to misdiagnosis and inadequate treatment for individuals from marginalised communities. These biases continue to perpetuate disparities and inequities in mental health care, echoing the racial prejudices of early psychologists.

Efforts to Dismantle Biases:

Modern psychology recognises the imperative need to dismantle these biases. Efforts are being made to create culturally responsive services, promote diversity within the mental health workforce, and develop diagnostic tools and treatment approaches that respect and incorporates diverse cultural contexts.

1. **Culturally Conscious Services:** Recognizing the need for culturally conscious mental health care has led to developing services that are

attuned to the specific needs of individuals from various cultural backgrounds.

2. **Promoting Diversity:** Encouraging diversity within the mental health profession helps to bridge the gap between providers and patients, fostering trust and understanding.

3. **Educational Reforms:** Incorporating cultural consciousness training in educational curricula for mental health professionals is essential to challenge and eradicate the biases inherited from the field's early days.

The ideologies of early psychological pioneers have had a lasting impact on the field, reflecting and reinforcing racial and gender biases. Understanding this dark history is essential to recognise the preferences that influence current mental health care practices. Through awareness, education, and a commitment to inclusivity and cultural consciousness, psychology can move towards a more equitable and just system that addresses the mental health needs of all individuals, regardless of their racial or ethnic background.

Shining a Light on the Dark Corners of Psychology is not merely an exercise in the historical examination. It is a call to action. It urges mental health professionals and society to critically examine how these enduring biases shape our understanding and treatment of mental health and commit to a path of reform, inclusivity, and cultural consciousness. In doing so, we can create a mental health care system that truly serves the needs and well-being of all its members, regardless of race, ethnicity, or gender.

Illuminating Thought-Terminating Clichés and Their Impact on Black Mental Health: A Call for Allies

Understanding the current state of Black mental health in the UK and globally involves an examination of the intricate mechanisms that perpetuate racial bias. Among these are thought-terminating clichés – emotionally potent phrases that halt critical thought and inhibit meaningful discourse on white supremacy and racism.

Thought-Terminating Clichés: A Closer Look

- **"Reverse Racism":** This cliché distracts from the systemic problem of white supremacy, proposing a false equivalence. *Example: "Why isn't there a White History Month? That's reverse racism!"* As someone often asked by white individuals, "Can black people be racist?" In return, I challenge this by asking, "Is there a racist word I can use against you or any racial discrimination you face due to the colour of your skin?"

If such a word does exist, does it carry the same historical weight, the same legacy of oppression, violence, and systemic discrimination? The words used as racial slurs against Black people are seeped in centuries of slavery, segregation, and subjugation. They are more than just derogatory terms; they represent a long history of racial hatred, deep-seated prejudice, and emotional and psychological trauma passed down through generations. The magnitude and gravity of these words are entrenched in a context of power imbalance and dehumanisation that is incomparable to any word that can be wielded against the dominant racial group.

- **"We're Post-Racial"**: This cliché asserts that society has outgrown racial discrimination, undermining the ongoing reality of structural racism. *Example: "We had a black president, Obama, so how can racism still exist?"*

- **"Not All White People"**: This cliché seeks to separate individuals from the systemic issue of white supremacy. *Example: "I'm not part of the problem; I treat everyone equally."*

- **"Playing the Race Card"**: This cliché seeks to discredit claims of racism. *Example: "He's just playing the race card to get sympathy; it has nothing to do with racism."*

- "**Colorblindness":** The idea of "colourblindness" stifles discussions about racial disparities. *Example: "I don't see colour, so I can't be racist."*

- **"All Lives Matter"**: This cliché often derails conversations about racial injustice. *Example: "Why focus on Black Lives Matter? Shouldn't all lives matter?"*

- **"I'm Not Racist Because I Have a Black Friend"**: This cliché attempts to dismiss accusations of personal racism. *Example: "I can't be racist; my best friend is black!"*

This dialogue illustrates how thought-terminating clichés are often used as a shield to avoid deep and uncomfortable conversations about race. By recognising and challenging these clichés, we can unravel the complexities of racism and engage in meaningful dialogue that fosters understanding and empathy.

The Shadow of History and the Dawn of Change: A Comprehensive Look at Black Mental Health in the UK Today

The footprints of psychology's founders, from Freud's essentialist notions of race to Jung's Eurocentric perspectives to Galton's eugenicist ideologies, still echo through the annals of psychology. These historical biases have engendered stereotypes, bolstered racial hierarchies, and alienated non-European communities, profoundly shaping the current narrative and treatment of Black mental health in the UK.

Today's challenges are not isolated incidents; they are the legacy of historical prejudice and Eurocentric supremacy. Current research by notable organisations such as the NHS, Mental Health Foundation and Mind illustrates the depth of these issues:

1. **Profound Inequality in Mental Health Care Access and Quality**: Socioeconomic disparities, including poverty and unemployment, disproportionately impact Black communities, leading to elevated mental illness rates. Despite these adversities, Black

individuals are 40% less likely to access talking therapies, indicating a stark inequality in cognitive healthcare accessibility and quality.

2. **Overrepresentation of Black Individuals in Mental Health Detentions**: Black individuals are more than four times as likely to be detained under the Mental Health Act than their white counterparts, highlighting a systemic failure to manage mental health crises in Black communities.

3. **Persistent Pathologization of Blackness**: There's a 6.8 times higher likelihood of Black men receiving a schizophrenia diagnosis than White men, revealing the lingering racial bias in mental health diagnoses.

4. **Barriers to Access to Mental Health Services**: While experiencing higher mental illness rates, only 6.2% of Black adults in England utilise mental health services compared to 13.3% of White adults. Factors like stigma, discrimination, and lack of culturally sensitive services contribute to these barriers, painting a picture of a mental healthcare system failing to serve Black communities effectively.

5. **Low Success and High Dropout Rates**: Therapy dropout rates are higher among Black individuals with lower success rates. These disparities can be attributed to a lack of cultural consciousness in therapeutic interventions, experiences of microaggressions within the

therapeutic environment, or cultural mismatches between therapists and clients.

6. **Mental Health Impacts of Racism and Experiences of Racism, Including Racial Trauma:** Racism significantly impacts Black individuals' mental health, creating a complex trauma often overlooked or misunderstood by culturally unconscious therapists. Racial trauma can increase the risk of mental health disorders, aggravate existing condition symptoms, and lead to higher stress and anxiety levels. Racial trauma may include microaggressions, racial harassment, racial violence, institutional racism, and the historical and intergenerational transmission of trauma. Culturally conscious therapy is needed to recognise and address this unique form of trauma that constitutes a significant, yet often overlooked, determinant of mental health disparities in Black communities.

These sobering realities are deeply rooted in psychology's colonial ideologies and the systemic biases they've fostered. They've cemented power dynamics between colonisers and the colonised, resulting in a mental healthcare landscape steeped in historical prejudice.

Nonetheless, a beacon of change is on the horizon. Acknowledging these disparities is the initial step, but the real journey is actively working to dismantle the deeply ingrained racial biases. The path forward demands a mental healthcare system that is accessible, culturally sensitive, and unchained from historical racial discrimination.

Understanding the current state of Black mental health in the UK is an intricate task, calling for a critical examination of the deeply rooted biases embedded in psychology's foundations. Now, more than ever, it's time to illuminate these dark corners and forge a path towards a future where mental healthcare respects and honours all individuals' diverse identities and experiences.

Overcoming Thought-Terminating Clichés: The Role of Allies

Recognition and confrontation of thought-terminating clichés in discussions about racial bias and white supremacy are crucial steps towards their dismantling. However, the work doesn't stop there. Allies - individuals from dominant racial groups - have an essential role.

History has shown us that no movement for equality and justice between a dominating majority and a minority ever achieved its goals without the support of allies. From the abolition of slavery to the suffragettes, gay rights, and the fight against apartheid, allies were crucial in these movements. As beneficiaries of inherent privileges, allies must actively engage in anti-racist practices. Silence or passivity serves only to perpetuate systemic racism and uphold white supremacy. By using their voices to amplify those of the marginalised, they contribute to significant change.

The importance of cultural consciousness in this journey is profound. Understanding diverse cultural experiences, acknowledging historical contexts, and validating the experiences of marginalised communities can equip us to effectively address systemic biases, paving the way towards a more equitable mental healthcare system.

In the next chapter, we will delve deeper into the role of allies and cultural consciousness in dismantling systemic biases and transforming mental healthcare. Through critical thinking, awareness, and cultural consciousness, we can counter the effects of thought-terminating clichés and shape a mental healthcare landscape that respects and honours diverse identities and experiences. It is a journey towards a future where conversations about race, racism, and mental health are navigated with nuance, compassion, and understanding, unrestricted by clichéd rhetoric.

A Personal and Professional Journey: Cultivating Cultural Consciousness in Mental Health Care

As a Black individual determined to seek therapy, I had overcome countless barriers to find myself seated in a stark, uninviting box room within my college. The room was far from the stereotype of a warm, welcoming therapist's office. Its harsh lighting was unforgiving, and its scant furnishings included a ticking clock, a nondescript table, two utilitarian chairs, and a lonely box of tissues. A far cry from the comforting ambience one might imagine for a place of healing.

The therapist to whom I'd been assigned, Holly, was a middle-aged white woman. Despite the sterile surroundings, her professional demeanour offered a semblance of normality. However, a lingering unease pulsed through me, nurtured by societal stigmas, racial stereotypes, and the inherent disparities in access to mental health care.

Buoyed by a hopeful spirit, I was eager to challenge these barriers to prove that therapy wasn't merely a luxury for the privileged but a universal right. However, as I learned, additional challenges lay ahead, invisible yet deeply entrenched within the system meant to aid healing.

My passion for psychology, usually a source of strength, altered the dynamic in the room. I noticed a change in Holly's posture, a retreat into the safety of her chair as I shared my thoughts. Her response, unexpected and disconcerting, sliced through my enthusiasm. "I sense aggression from you," she stated. Her words echoed the unfounded stereotype so often projected onto Black men in our society. Flustered, I hastened to explain myself, hoping to dismantle her misconstrued perceptions. Yet, the stain of that label, 'aggressive,' had already seeped in.

In the following experiences with other white therapists, attempts to explore my experiences with racial discrimination were met with dismissive cliches. "We're all part of the human race, aren't we?" They countered, their words nullifying my lived experiences and perpetuating the racial stereotypes I was there to address. Disoriented and dejected, I left each session feeling unseen and invalidated.

As my journey towards becoming a therapist progressed, I recognised my experiences as symptomatic of systemic racism embedded in the fabric of mental health care - from curriculum and diagnostic criteria to treatment approaches and the evident lack of diversity and cultural consciousness.

This realisation stirred a potent desire to challenge the status quo and cultivate a landscape where mental health care recognises and respects the experiences and needs of marginalised communities.

Today, in my practice as a therapist, I commit myself to create a safe and validating environment for every individual, irrespective of their background. To challenge unconscious and conscious biases, continually learn and unlearn, listen intently to my client's stories, and develop treatment plans that respect their cultural values.

Cultivating cultural consciousness is a shared journey. It's an ongoing process that requires the commitment of mental health professionals, policymakers, researchers, and the wider community. We must unite to dismantle systemic barriers, increase diversity within the field, and ensure that diagnostic criteria and treatment approaches reflect diverse experiences.

By embracing cultural consciousness, we can move beyond the limitations of the past and build an inclusive, empowering, and effective mental health care system. This journey is challenging, but it's also a hopeful one. A journey towards a future where mental health care is a beacon of hope and healing for every individual, regardless of race, culture, or background.

Let's undertake this transformative journey together and strive for a brighter future for mental health care.

Chapter 1 Key Points:

1. **Historical Context of Racial Bias:** This chapter begins by exploring the historical bias entrenched in psychology, considering how early pioneers like Freud, Jung, and Galton have influenced perceptions and treatment of Black mental health. Their predominantly Eurocentric ideologies perpetuated racial hierarchies, marginalised non-European communities, and continue to influence today's mental healthcare landscape significantly.

2. **Enduring Legacy of Biases:** Rather than simply relics of the past, these historical biases continue to manifest as enduring issues within today's mental healthcare system. This enduring legacy presents disparities in mental health care access and quality, overrepresentation of Black individuals in mental health detentions, the persistent pathologisation of Blackness, and existing barriers to mental health services.

3. **Mental Health Disparities:** The chapter emphasises stark disparities in mental health outcomes between Black and white populations in the UK, substantiated by research from reputable organisations such as the NHS, Mental Health Foundation, and Mind. This section explores numerous issues,

including socioeconomic determinants of mental health, frequent misdiagnoses, low success and high dropout rates in therapy, and the pervasive impacts of racism on mental health.

4. **Impacts of Racism and Discrimination:** The narrative places a strong emphasis on the detrimental effects of racism and discrimination on the mental health of Black individuals, including higher risks of developing mental health disorders, exacerbation of existing condition symptoms, and elevated stress and anxiety levels.

5. **Urgent Need for Systemic Change:** This chapter underscores the urgent need for systemic change within the mental healthcare system to address these deeply ingrained racial biases effectively. It advocates for a future mental healthcare system that is accessible, culturally conscious, and free from historical racial preferences, necessitating a proactive and determined approach to dismantling these entrenched biases.

6. **The Crucial Role of Allies:** The chapter introduces the concept of allies and highlights their vital role in achieving racial justice and equality. It underscores that historical movements for freedom or rights, such as the abolition of slavery, suffrage, gay rights and marriage equality, and the end of apartheid, all relied significantly on the support of allies from dominant groups.

7. **Emphasizing Cultural Consciousness and Countering Thought-Terminating Clichés:** **The** chapter culminates with an emphasis on cultivating cultural consciousness and challenging thought-terminating clichés – phrases that hinder critical thinking and suppress discourse on racism and white supremacy. These crucial tools are instrumental in shaping a more equitable, inclusive approach to mental healthcare.

In the realm of mental health, breaking the silence and challenging biases are the keys to transformation. Embracing mental health is a collective endeavour where empathy guides our steps, and cultural consciousness empowers us. Let us rise above misconceptions, liberate ourselves from shame, and foster well-being for all.

Jarell Bempong.

Chapter 2

Unpacking Biases and Fostering Cultural Consciousness: Empowering Individuals

Embracing Mental Health: Overcoming Stereotypes and Finding Liberation

Born in the bustling city of London; my life took an unexpected turn when, at around age twelve, my parents decided to move us to Ghana. This change provoked me to question my narrow understanding of mental health, a view heavily influenced by cultural misconceptions and societal biases. My only reference for mental health was "abodamfoo," a term synonymous with "mad" or mentally unwell people, depicting a bleak picture of individuals cast aside and stigmatised by society.

Within my community, discussions on mental health were non-existent, marked by a shroud of silence and misunderstanding. Mental health was equated to a problematic existence – confusion, poor hygiene, humiliation, and sometimes violence. This distorted viewpoint created a barrier that obstructed our ability to recognise and handle mental health issues. We believed that silent suffering was the only option, given the prevailing cultural norms against discussing personal issues or airing family matters.

My journey was fraught with challenges. As a dyslexic student, I faced struggles in education that often left me feeling defeated. Furthermore, coming to terms with my sexual identity in a society deeply rooted in religious beliefs, superstitions, and homophobia proved daunting. These challenges, coupled with unresolved childhood trauma from a broken family and lack of support, unresolved childhood trauma from a broken family, and lack of support further complicated my struggles.

At eighteen, I returned to the UK for freedom from the oppressive atmosphere I experienced in Ghana. I didn't realise that undiagnosed and treatable mental health conditions silently shaped my life. Unaware of these underlying issues, I continued to suffer silently, oblivious that help was available.

However, my life took a decisive turn when I encountered a counselling course. In the safety of the counselling room, I met Holly, a mental health professional who I hoped would offer empathy and understanding. Unfortunately, this encounter was my first experience with racism and stereotypes within a mental health context, which was disheartening.

Despite the hurdles, my resolve to understand mental health deepened. I embarked on a journey of self-discovery, challenging cultural stigmas and breaking the silence. I reclaimed my power for myself and others trapped within the confines of societal prejudice.

I decided to challenge mental health stigma within our communities by sharing my story and advocating for change. I became a symbol of hope, fostering self-acceptance, understanding, and growth. By challenging stereotypes and promoting open dialogues, I realised we could collectively reshape the mental health narrative and build a society that prioritises our well-being.

Today, I stand as a testament to the human spirit's resilience and the importance of recognising mental health. My journey has taught me the value of breaking down cultural barriers, seeking support, and promoting a society that accepts mental health as a crucial part of overall well-being.

Through my journey of self-discovery, I found my voice and purpose—to empower others, raise awareness, and advocate for a mental health care system that acknowledges diverse human experiences. By challenging stereotypes and promoting inclusivity, we can create a society where individuals are liberated from the shackles of silence and thrive.

Unveiling Mental Health Biases: Challenging Assumptions and Fostering Personal Well-Being

In mental health, biases and assumptions can significantly impact an individual's well-being. Society often holds certain beliefs and stereotypes about mental health, which can lead to misconceptions, stigma, and barriers to seeking support. This chapter explores the biases and assumptions that individuals may hold regarding mental health and their profound effects on personal well-being. By challenging these biases and fostering a more inclusive and empathetic understanding, we can create a supportive environment that promotes mental well-being for all.

Biases and Assumptions:

1. **Stigma and Shame:** One common bias surrounding mental health is the stigma of seeking help. Many individuals believe that acknowledging mental health struggles is a sign of weakness or failure, leading to feelings of shame. This bias can prevent individuals from seeking the necessary support and exacerbate health issues.
2. **Lack of Understanding:** Biases and assumptions can stem from a lack of understanding or awareness about mental health. Misconceptions about mental illnesses may lead individuals to believe that those struggling with mental health are "crazy" or "unstable." This lack of understanding perpetuates stereotypes and hinders empathy and support for those in need.
3. **Minimization and Invalidating Experiences:** Some biases may trivialise mental health struggles, dismissing them as mood swings or attention-seeking behaviour. This depreciation can invalidate experiences, which prevents them from receiving the support they need and contributes to feelings of isolation and distress.
4. **Cultural and Gender Biases:** Biases related to culture and gender can also influence perceptions of mental health. For example, certain cultures may stigmatise mental health issues, viewing them as a personal failing rather than a medical condition. Gender biases may result in expectations for individuals to

suppress emotions or discourage seeking help, particularly among men.

Impact on Personal Well-being:

The prevailing prejudices and misconceptions about mental health can profoundly impact personal well-being.

1. **Delayed Help-seeking**: The stigma and embarrassment often attached to mental health issues can deter individuals from seeking necessary assistance promptly. This delay can exacerbate symptoms, heighten distress and considerably undermine overall well-being.
2. **Social Isolation:** Prejudices and preconceived notions can alienate those grappling with mental health issues by constructing barriers to open conversations and understanding. The apprehension of judgment and rejection may compel individuals to withdraw from their support systems, heightening feelings of loneliness and isolation.
3. **Internalised Self-stigma:** Individuals risk developing self-stigma when they absorb and internalise societal prejudices and stereotypes. They may perceive themselves as weak, defective, or unworthy of support, which can harm self-esteem, confidence, and overall well-being.
4. **Limited Treatment Options:** Prejudices and misconceptions can curtail the range and effectiveness of available treatment options.

Misunderstandings about mental health may lead individuals to depend solely on self-help methods or alternative therapies, potentially bypassing evidence-based treatments that could significantly enhance their well-being.

Promoting Personal Well-being:

To advance personal well-being and confront biases about mental health, specific actions must be taken:

Education and Awareness: Enhancing education and raising awareness about mental health can dispel misconceptions and diminish stigma. We can shape a more informed and empathetic society by fostering open conversations and disseminating accurate information.

Empathy and Understanding: Encouraging compassion and understanding towards those dealing with mental health issues is paramount. Active listening, validating experiences, and extending support can help dismantle prejudices and cultivate an ethos of compassion and acceptance.

Inclusive Language and Narratives: Language plays a crucial role in shaping perceptions. Utilising inclusive language that shuns stigmatising labels or derogatory terms aids in creating a supportive environment. Promoting diverse narratives and experiences helps challenge assumptions and encourage inclusivity.

Accessible and Equitable Services: It's imperative to ensure that mental health services are accessible and equitable. Eliminating barriers such as cost, location, and cultural consciousness can aid individuals in overcoming biases and accessing the support they need for their well-being.

Confronting biases and misconceptions about mental health can lead to a society that values and prioritises personal well-being. Through education, empathy, inclusive language, and equitable services, we can counteract the detrimental effects of biases and cultivate a supportive environment where everyone can access the mental health support they deserve. We can bolster personal well-being and dismantle the barriers preventing individuals from leading fulfilling lives.

Decoding Mental Health: Confronting Biases and Cultivating Wellness

Within the sanctum of therapy, an environment meant to encourage healing and growth, biases can unintentionally obscure the path towards accurate understanding and connection. We delve into the profound effect of prejudice within therapeutic relationships, exploring the transformative journey of self-discovery and development for clients and therapists. The narrative unfolds through my personal experience as a client, where Holly's unintentional biases reveal hidden truths that linger beneath the surface of mental healthcare.

Looking back at the inaugural session with Holly, the profound impact of her latent biases is strikingly evident. As a mental health professional, I thought therapists were invulnerable to such sway, the epitome of impartiality and understanding. However, that session shattered my illusions, exposing the unsettling truth that therapists, too, can unconsciously entertain biases that can distort the therapeutic process.

As we embark on this journey of self-reflection and growth, we unravel the intricacies of biases in therapy. My transformation helps us delve into the complex interplay of assumptions, preconceptions, and societal influences shaping our therapeutic experiences. Armed with unwavering honesty, we confront discomforting realities and start to dismantle the barriers obstructing genuine connection and healing.

As clients and mental health professionals, we jointly explore the profound repercussions of biases within therapeutic relationships. We reveal the transformative power of self-awareness, shedding light on the prejudices that mould our thoughts, perceptions, and interactions. Embracing this journey of self-discovery and committing to perpetual learning, we aim to create an inclusive and empowering therapeutic environment where biases are acknowledged, confronted, and eliminated.

Biases, deeply embedded in our consciousness, can mould our thoughts, perceptions, and behaviours, often without our conscious realisation. Acknowledging and tackling these biases is crucial in nurturing a more inclusive and equitable society. Thus, we delve into practical strategies for individuals to recognise their preferences and proactively work towards eliminating them. Embarking on this transformative journey of self-reflection and growth, we can contribute towards a more unbiased world.

Battling Biases: Essential Strategies for Fostering Self-Awareness and Promoting Inclusivity:

Self-Reflection and Honest Examination: Unravelling self-reflection commences with an honest examination of our beliefs, attitudes, and behaviours. This process necessitates introspection and a readiness to confront uncomfortable truths about our biases, asking ourselves challenging questions and welcoming feedback from others.

Education and Exposure: Enlightenment about diverse cultures, identities, and experiences is essential for bias awareness and elimination. Actively seeking out information, engaging in conversations, and forming connections with people from diverse backgrounds provide valuable insights and foster empathy.

Mindfulness and Self-Awareness: Developing mindfulness and self-awareness allows us to identify biases as they surface in our thoughts, emotions, and reactions. A heightened self-awareness empowers us to pause, reflect, and opt for more inclusive and equitable responses.

Challenging Assumptions and Stereotypes: Biases often stem from assumptions and stereotypes we entertain about specific groups. Actively questioning these assumptions and seeking evidence to counter them is crucial for bias elimination.

Seeking Diverse Perspectives: Engaging with diverse perspectives is fundamental for bias awareness and elimination. Actively seeking and listening to voices that challenge our beliefs helps dismantle stereotypes and broaden our understanding.

Fostering Empathy and Encouraging Perspective-Taking: Cultivating empathy and mastering perspective-taking empowers us to transcend our personal experiences and gain insight into the realities of others. By fostering empathy, we facilitate connection and set the stage for effectively eliminating biases.

Acting: Awareness alone is inadequate; action is necessary to eliminate biases. This requires actively challenging biased behaviours, language, and systems, advocating for policy changes, and supporting initiatives that promote diversity, equity, and inclusion.

Becoming aware of our biases and actively working to eliminate them is a transformative and ongoing journey. It requires humility, self-reflection, education, empathy, and the courage to challenge ingrained beliefs. By embracing this process, we can contribute to a more inclusive and equitable society where biases no longer dictate our thoughts and actions. Let us commence this journey together, recognising the power of personal change to shape a better future for all.

The Future of Mental Health: Cultural Consciousness Revolutionising Therapy

Embracing Diversity: Benefits and Key Steps to Implementing Cultural Consciousness in Therapy

Modern psychotherapy, grappling with inherent racism, opens a path towards the potential solution of Culturally Conscious therapy. This method aims to eradicate harmful biases and deliver effective therapeutic care for individuals across diverse cultural backgrounds. This inclusive, equitable approach recognises and respects all individuals' unique experiences and needs, irrespective of their cultural identity.

Cultural Consciousness: Embracing Diversity and Cultural Understanding

Cultural consciousness is recognising, appreciating, and understanding diverse cultural perspectives, beliefs, values, and experiences. Its cultivation promotes inclusivity, equity, and meaningful connections in mental health, the workplace, and broader society.

Cultural Consciousness and the Fufu Adventure:

Let me share a hilarious example that illustrates cultural consciousness in action. Imagine a day in Ghana when my stepdad found himself ravenously hungry, and the only available food was a traditional Ghanaian dish called fufu. Fufu is a unique delicacy made from cassava and plantains, cooked, and pounded into a smooth and sticky consistency.

Fufu is different from what you would call a universally appealing dish. Its sticky and gummy texture can be pretty challenging for the uninitiated. Nevertheless, in a moment of cultural curiosity, my mom kindly offered my stepdad some fufu. With a mix of trepidation and hunger in his eyes, he hesitantly agreed to try it.

My stepdad experienced a taste and texture sensation with just one mouthful of fufu. As he chewed on the sticky fufu, his facial expressions were priceless. We could not help but burst into laughter at the sight of his humorous struggle to handle the unique texture of the dish.

In between bouts of laughter, we asked, "Do you like it?" With a mischievous glint in his eye, my stepdad managed to utter, "That was enough for me!" It was clear that while he embraced the cultural adventure by trying the fufu, one mouthful was more than enough to satisfy his curiosity.

Although my stepdad did not develop a newfound love for fufu, that one comical experience exemplified cultural consciousness. He embraced the opportunity to engage with a diverse cultural practice, even if the taste and texture didn't align with his preferences. His willingness to try and light-hearted reaction created a memorable moment that fostered understanding and appreciation for Ghanaian traditions.

This funny fufu story highlights the importance of cultural consciousness in breaking down barriers and embracing diversity. It reminds us that even a single bite can offer insight into a different culture and that willingness to step outside our comfort zones can cultivate understanding and build bridges of connection.

Cultural consciousness is a continuous journey of learning, unlearning biases, and cultivating respect for the richness of human experiences. By actively seeking knowledge, embracing cultural differences, and engaging in meaningful interactions, we can contribute to a more inclusive and harmonious world, all while sharing a good laugh.

So, let us savour the hilarity and embrace cultural consciousness, one mouthful at a time.

The Power of Understanding: Unpacking Cultural Consciousness and Its Role in Mental Health

Cultural consciousness can transform mental health by fostering inclusivity and equity. Therapists who embrace cultural consciousness create a safe and welcoming space for patients from various backgrounds. This involves considering cultural factors such as values, beliefs, and practises and understanding how they influence an individual's mental health and overall well-being.

One of the primary benefits of cultural consciousness in mental health is its ability to bridge the gap between patients and therapists. By acknowledging and valuing a patient's cultural background, therapists establish a stronger connection and build trust. This is particularly important for clients from underrepresented groups who may have encountered stigma or discrimination within the mental health system.

Furthermore, cultural consciousness helps reduce bias and enhances cultural competence among therapists. By gaining a deeper understanding of diverse cultures, therapists become more aware of their preferences and can develop more effective approaches to collaborating with patients from diverse backgrounds. This, in turn, leads to better treatment outcomes and fosters a more favourable therapeutic relationship.

In addition to improving the therapeutic relationship, cultural consciousness enables more effective treatment. By understanding the cultural factors contributing to a patient's mental health concerns, therapists can develop targeted and personalised treatment plans tailored to the individual's needs. This approach promotes better outcomes and a more positive experience for the patient.

Building Bridges and Breaking Barriers: The Critical Need for Cultural Consciousness in Today's Diverse World

Cultural consciousness is not limited to therapy and mental health alone. In today's interconnected world, where people from diverse cultural backgrounds frequently interact, embracing cultural consciousness is vital in all aspects of life. It allows individuals to understand and appreciate the differences and similarities among various cultural groups, fostering greater understanding and respect for diverse perspectives and experiences.

Cultural consciousness helps to avoid misunderstandings, stereotyping, and discrimination based on cultural differences, leading to stronger relationships and more effective communication with people from diverse cultural backgrounds. Moreover, in contexts such as business or diplomacy, being culturally conscious is crucial for success and effective collaboration across cultures.

Beyond Borders: Exploring the Many Spaces Where Cultural Consciousness Can Transform Lives

The impact of cultural consciousness extends far beyond therapy and mental health. In an increasingly globalised world, individuals must embrace cultural consciousness in all areas of life. Understanding and valuing diverse perspectives can create more inclusive and equitable environments in the workplace, educational institutions, or social settings.

In the workplace, cultural consciousness fosters effective communication, increases creativity, and enhances problem-solving. Collaboration among individuals from diverse backgrounds brings unique perspectives, leading to innovative ideas and solutions.

Cultural consciousness promotes an inclusive learning environment within educational institutions where all students feel valued and respected. Teachers who incorporate cultural consciousness into their curriculum help students learn about diverse cultures and better understand the world, fostering empathy and creating a more inclusive school community.

In social settings, cultural consciousness helps individuals develop more meaningful relationships with people from diverse cultures. Being open to different perspectives and understanding cultural practices builds bridges and forms deeper connections with individuals who may have been perceived as "other" previously.

Cultivating Cultural Consciousness: Recognising the Many Opportunities for Inclusion and Understanding in Our Daily Lives

Cultural consciousness is not limited to specific settings or times; it is a mindset that can be applied to all aspects of life. Countless opportunities exist to recognise and embrace diverse cultural perspectives, from the workplace to the classroom and social interactions.

In the workplace, being culturally conscious involves acknowledging and valuing the diversity of colleagues, customers, and clients. This includes being open to different ideas and ways of working and being mindful of cultural practices or beliefs that may impact the work environment. Creating a more inclusive and equitable workplace environment fosters a sense of value and respect for everyone.

Cultural consciousness involves incorporating diverse cultural perspectives into lessons and discussions in educational institutions. Teachers can develop a curriculum that includes various voices and experiences while being mindful of cultural practices or beliefs that may influence students' learning. By doing so, students better understand the world and develop greater empathy and understanding for those with diverse backgrounds.

In social interactions, being culturally conscious means being open to different ideas and ways of living. It requires mindfulness of cultural practices or beliefs that may differ from one's own and respect for the cultural heritage of those around them. By fostering respect and understanding, individuals can build relationships based on mutual respect and gain a deeper appreciation for diverse cultures.

To be culturally conscious is to appreciate the richness and variety of human experience. By doing so, mental health professionals may build a system that better meets the requirements of all their patients in terms of accessibility, fairness, and compassion. Moreover, raising one's level of cultural awareness in every facet of life aids in dismantling stereotypes, developing greater empathy, and advancing understanding among people of various cultural origins. Understanding and appreciating one another's cultural backgrounds can build a society where everyone feels included and respected.

Culturally Conscious Therapy: Embracing Diversity for Authentic Healing

As I author this book, my thoughts drift back to that significant encounter that deeply impacted my understanding of cultural consciousness in therapy. It was pivotal when I was stereotyped as aggressive during a session with Holly, my first therapist. Although I have touched on this encounter before, its repercussions continue to resonate within me.

As I poured my heart out, passionately expressing my thoughts and emotions in that therapy room, I noticed a subtle shift in Holly's demeanour. The unmistakable discomfort in her eyes betrayed her perception of me as aggressive instead of recognising my passion and intensity for what they indeed were.

At that time, I struggled with how to respond. I felt an innate urge to defend myself and explain that my words were fuelled by passion, not aggression. Yet I found myself grappling with the weight of stereotypes projected onto me, momentarily unsure how to challenge them effectively.

However, with the passage of time and a deeper exploration of cultural consciousness, I have gained invaluable insights and a profound sense of empowerment. Today, as an expert in this field, I approach this encounter with renewed purpose and clarity.

In this book, I aim to draw upon my personal journey and professional expertise to guide therapists and clients in cultivating cultural consciousness within the therapeutic space. Together, we will embark on a transformative journey, challenging biases, dismantling stereotypes, and fostering a deeper understanding of cultural nuances.

By delving into practical strategies and effective communication techniques, we can foster an inclusive and equitable therapeutic environment that honours the diversity of cultural expressions and paves the way for authentic healing and growth.

5 Levels of Cultural Consciousness: Moving from Unconscious/Ignorant to Conscious

Developing cultural consciousness is essential for fostering understanding, empathy, and inclusivity in a world of cultural diversity and interconnectedness. Developing cultural consciousness is vital to promoting understanding, compassion, and inclusivity in a world of cultural diversity and interconnectedness. Cultural consciousness encompasses a spectrum of awareness, from unconsciousness to cultural humility, representing different levels of knowledge and engagement with diverse cultures. This journey of cultural consciousness involves recognising the influence of cultural factors on human experiences, challenging biases and assumptions, and actively striving for cultural competence and humility. By exploring the various levels of cultural consciousness, we embark on a transformative exploration of personal growth and societal change, aiming to build bridges across cultures and create a more harmonious and equitable world.

1. **Unconscious/Ignorant:** At this level, individuals operate without awareness or recognition of the importance of cultural factors in everyday interactions and understanding. They may need to gain knowledge about diverse cultural backgrounds, understand the impact of culture on human experiences, and overlook the influence of social and contextual factors. Individuals at this

level are more prone to making assumptions based on their cultural perspectives, which may inadvertently perpetuate stereotypes and biases.

2. **Emerging Awareness:** Individuals at this level start to recognise cultural differences and their potential impact on interactions and relationships. They may acknowledge the need to consider cultural factors but possess limited knowledge or understanding of specific cultural nuances. There is a growing realisation that cultural competence is vital in communication and building connections. Individuals begin to seek out educational opportunities to enhance their cultural awareness.

3. **Cultural Sensitivity**: At this stage, individuals actively cultivate cultural sensitivity. They engage in ongoing self-reflection, examining their biases and assumptions and seeking to understand their cultural lenses. They try to learn about diverse cultural backgrounds, traditions, and belief systems. Individuals at this level strive to approach others with an open mind, respecting and valuing different perspectives and experiences.

4. **Cultural Competence:** Individuals at this level demonstrate an elevated level of cultural competence in their everyday interactions. They possess a deep understanding of the cultural factors that influence human experiences, recognise the diversity within cultural groups, and are skilled at navigating cultural complexities. They

actively engage in cross-cultural communication, adapt their communication styles to be inclusive and respectful, and are sensitive to potential misunderstandings. Individuals at this level actively work to address power imbalances, promote inclusivity, and foster equity in their interactions and communities.

5. **Cultural Humility:** The highest level of cultural consciousness is characterised by cultural humility. Individuals at this stage approach each interaction with a genuine desire to learn from and respect the unique cultural experiences of others. They recognise the limitations of their knowledge and continuously seek to expand their cultural understanding. They engage in ongoing self-reflection and actively seek feedback from others to ensure culturally responsive interactions. Individuals at this level acknowledge the importance of lifelong learning, vigorously challenge systemic inequities, and advocate for the inclusion and empowerment of marginalised communities in all aspects of life.

As individuals progress from unconsciousness to cultural humility, they can better understand the influence of culture on human experiences and interactions. Achieving higher levels of cultural consciousness requires ongoing self-reflection, education, and a commitment to challenging and dismantling systemic barriers perpetuating societal disparities and inequities. By fostering cultural consciousness, individuals can contribute to a more inclusive and harmonious society where diverse perspectives and experiences are valued and respected.

Empowering Strategies: Nurturing Cultural Consciousness in Therapy and Beyond

Starting your journey towards cultural awareness can seem like a big task, but remember that even the longest journey begins with a single step. This critical path requires understanding, empathy, and a solid commitment to creating inclusive environments. As we move through our diverse world, we must arm ourselves with the right tools to challenge biases, break down stereotypes, and encourage inclusivity.

To help you on this journey, here are some simple and effective strategies that you can use not only in therapy sessions but also in your everyday life:

1. **Educate Yourself:** Education is a powerful tool for promoting inclusivity and challenging discriminatory practices. Take the initiative to educate yourself about diverse cultures, customs, traditions, and histories. For example, you can read books by authors from diverse backgrounds, watch documentaries highlighting the experiences of marginalised communities, and engage in online resources that provide accurate and varied perspectives. By expanding your knowledge, you can develop a deeper understanding of cultural diversity and challenge stereotypes and biases.

2. **Examine Your Biases:** Awareness of your biases and assumptions is essential. Take the time to reflect on your beliefs and attitudes towards diverse cultures and communities. Challenge any stereotypes or prejudices you may hold and strive to replace them with accurate information and empathy. Engage in self-reflection and consider how your biases may impact your interactions with others. For instance, you can ask yourself questions like, "What preconceived notions do I have about certain cultures?" or "How can I challenge these biases and foster a more inclusive mindset?"

3. **Engage in Meaningful Dialogue:** Dialogue promotes inclusivity and challenges discriminatory practices. Actively seek out opportunities to engage with individuals from diverse backgrounds. Listen attentively to their stories, experiences, and perspectives. Ask questions respectfully and approach conversations with an open mind. By fostering dialogue, you can learn from others, challenge your assumptions, and build bridges of understanding. For example, you can participate in community forums or join online discussion groups where people from diverse backgrounds share their perspectives and engage in constructive conversations.

4. **Be mindful of language and behaviours:** Language and behaviours can significantly impact promoting inclusivity or perpetuating discrimination. Be aware of the words you use and the actions you take. Avoid making derogatory comments or jokes that reinforce stereotypes or belittle others. Respect cultural norms around personal space, directness, and hierarchy. Be open to feedback and willing to adjust to ensure your language and behaviour are inclusive and respectful. For instance, you can consciously use gender-neutral language or learn how to correctly pronounce and address individuals' names.

5. **Advocate for Inclusion:** Actively advocating for inclusion and equality in your personal and professional spheres. Speak up against discriminatory practices and biases when you witness them. Use your voice to promote awareness and educate others about the importance of inclusivity. Support organisations and initiatives that work towards creating a more equitable society. By becoming an advocate for inclusion, you can inspire change and encourage others to challenge discriminatory practices. For example, you can participate in local community meetings or join advocacy groups that address social justice and inclusivity issues.

6. **Foster Inclusive Spaces:** Create safe and inclusive spaces for people of all cultures to express themselves and feel valued. Encourage diversity in your social circles, workplace, and community. Celebrate cultural events and festivals, promoting cross-cultural understanding and appreciation. By fostering inclusive spaces, you can help to create a sense of belonging and equality.

7. **Act:** Advocating for inclusivity requires more than passive understanding; it necessitates action. Engage in activities and initiatives that promote social justice and challenge discriminatory practices. Volunteer with organisations that support marginalised communities. Use your skills and resources to uplift underrepresented voices and contribute to positive change.

Final Remarks: The Continuous Journey Towards Inclusivity and Cultural Consciousness

In summary, the fight for inclusivity and the battle against discriminatory practices is a responsibility we all bear. Nurturing cultural consciousness is a complex task. Instead, it demands a relentless commitment to lifelong learning and growth. Educating ourselves, confronting our biases, engaging in significant conversations, being aware of our language and behaviours, advocating for inclusion, creating inclusive spaces, and taking meaningful action can trigger positive transformations in our communities and society.

I invite everyone to seize this opportunity to serve as a champion of inclusivity and aid in shaping a more fair and equal world. Our exploration of this vital journey is far from over. As we transition into the next chapter, we shift our focus towards a more specific audience - mental health professionals - and consider practical tools and strategies they can use to provide culturally conscious care.

Our understanding of the pervasive and long-lasting effects of racial trauma on Black individuals and cultural minorities, alongside recognising the unique challenges these communities face when seeking mental health care, compels us to press for progress. As we delve deeper, we will uncover how a commitment to self-reflection and cultural consciousness can help us deliver tailored, effective therapeutic services and catalyse transformative healing and positive change in these communities. Stay tuned as we continue this critical journey together.

Chapter 2 Key Points:

1. The Journey of Transformation: The chapter began with a personal anecdote emphasising the importance of cultural consciousness in therapy. My experience highlighted the importance of understanding and correctly interpreting the nuances of artistic expression within a therapeutic environment.

2. Levels of Cultural Consciousness: A spectrum of cultural consciousness was outlined, ranging from unconscious/ignorant to cultural humility. It emphasised the need to journey from a lack of awareness to active engagement and humility in understanding cultural differences. This transformation is crucial in challenging biases, dismantling stereotypes, and fostering a deeper understanding of cultural nuances.

3. Promoting Inclusivity and Challenging Discriminatory Practices: Individual responsibility was emphasised to foster and challenge discriminatory practices daily. This process necessitates continuous effort and a commitment to lifelong learning and growth.

4. Empowering Strategies for Cultivating Cultural Consciousness: A range of strategies was provided to cultivate cultural consciousness, including self-education, examining personal biases, engaging in meaningful dialogue, mindfulness of language and behaviour, active advocacy for inclusion, fostering inclusive spaces, and direct action.

5. The Role of Action: The chapter emphasised that advocacy for inclusivity and equity requires more than passive understanding or empathy; it necessitates action. Involvement in initiatives promoting social justice, volunteering with supportive organisations, and leveraging personal skills and resources to uplift underrepresented voices is critical for positive change.

"Cultural consciousness in mental health fosters individualized support for Black and minority communities. Through introspection and training, we catalyze transformative healing and change."

- Jarell Bempong

Chapter 3

Culturally Conscious Care

Improving Mental Health Care: Tailored Approaches for Black Communities and Other Cultural Minorities.

As a mental health professional, I am deeply committed to providing 1-on-1 therapy focusing on Black and cultural minority clients. This dedication stems from recognising Black individuals' unique challenges in accessing quality mental health care and the critical need for representation within therapeutic spaces. Black communities have long been underserved, experiencing significant disparities in mental health outcomes and limited access to culturally sensitive support. It is with extraordinary joy and a sense of purpose that I witness increasingly Black individuals benefiting from therapy and reclaiming their mental well-being.

The effects of racial trauma on black individuals cannot be understated. It encompasses various forms of trauma, including intergenerational, historical, childhood, and ongoing racial stressors. Intergenerational trauma refers to the transmission of trauma across generations resulting from the historical injustices endured by Black ancestors. This includes experiences of slavery, racial violence, and forced displacement, which continues to impact the collective psyche of Black communities. Historical trauma recognises the enduring effects of systemic oppression and racial discrimination on the mental health of Black individuals, stemming from events such as colonisation, segregation, and the civil rights movement.

Additionally, the daily experiences of racism, known as microaggressions, contribute to racial trauma. This subtle verbal, nonverbal, or environmental discrimination can be incredibly distressing and perpetuate a sense of otherness, invalidation, and marginalisation. Furthermore, institutional racism persists within education, healthcare, and criminal justice systems, exacerbating disparities and perpetuating inequities for Black individuals.

Addressing the multifaceted layers of racial trauma requires understanding the lived experiences and cultural nuances specific to Black clients. By recognising and validating these experiences, therapy becomes a haven where individuals can explore and heal from the impact of intergenerational trauma, historical trauma, microaggressions, and institutional racism. Within this therapeutic space, I aim to provide support, promote resilience, and empower Black individuals on their journey towards healing and self-discovery.

Moreover, successful mental health care for Black individuals extends beyond addressing trauma alone. Lifestyle determinants play a significant role in fostering overall well-being. This includes promoting self-care practices, healthy coping mechanisms, and community support. By integrating these elements into therapy, individuals can develop a comprehensive approach to mental health that considers their unique cultural backgrounds, values, and strengths.

In conclusion, as a mental health professional, I am driven by a profound commitment to providing 1-on-1 therapy that focuses on Black clients. By acknowledging and understanding the effects of racial trauma, including intergenerational trauma, historical trauma, microaggressions, and institutional racism, therapy becomes a transformative journey towards healing, resilience, and empowerment. I am deeply humbled and filled with joy when I witness more Black individuals benefiting from treatment, reclaiming their mental well-being, and embracing their inherent strengths. Together, we can create a future where mental health care is accessible, inclusive, and affirming for all.

Unleashing the Power of Cultural Consciousness.

In the ever-evolving field of mental health care, one fundamental truth stands resolute: no two individuals are exactly alike. We are complex beings shaped by a tapestry of experiences, identities, and cultural backgrounds. Recognising and embracing this diversity is an ethical imperative and a catalyst for transformative healing. Culturally conscious care is the cornerstone of empowering mental health professionals to navigate the intricacies of their clients' unique needs while fostering inclusivity, understanding, and positive change. This chapter delves into the practical tools and strategies mental health professionals can employ to provide culturally conscious care within their therapeutic practice, the broader workforce, and society.

Understanding Cultural Consciousness: A Multifaceted Approach.

Cultural consciousness goes beyond surface-level awareness; it involves a deep understanding and respect for the diverse cultures, beliefs, and values that shape individuals' lived experiences. It requires mental health professionals to navigate the complex interplay between cultural backgrounds and mental health, recognising how societal, historical, and systemic factors influence an individual's well-being. Mental health professionals must cultivate a solid foundation of knowledge, empathy, and humility to provide culturally conscious care.

1. **Self-Reflection and Awareness:** The Journey Begins Within The first step towards providing culturally conscious care lies in self-reflection and awareness. Mental health professionals must critically examine their biases, assumptions, and cultural lenses. This introspective journey enables them to uncover hidden prejudices, challenge ingrained stereotypes, and foster a genuine curiosity and openness towards diverse cultural perspectives. By engaging in ongoing self-reflection, mental health professionals can continuously refine their understanding of cultural dynamics and develop a greater capacity for empathy.

For example, a mental health professional may examine their implicit biases and reflect on how they might impact their interactions with clients from diverse cultural backgrounds. They may explore their cultural upbringing, values, and beliefs to understand better their cultural lens and how it may differ from their clients'. This self-awareness forms the foundation for culturally conscious care.

2. **Expanding Horizons with Cultural Consciousness Training:** Cultural consciousness extends beyond self-reflection, often necessitating the structure and expertise formal training offers. This training enriches participants with essential knowledge and skills to gracefully navigate the intricacies of cultural diversity. Such programs cover many topics, from cultural awareness and humility to intersectionality, norms, traditions, and the influence of historical contexts.

Participating in workshops, seminars, and continuing education programs is an impactful method for professionals to expand their cultural competence. This enriched understanding can enhance the quality of care provided to clients from diverse backgrounds. I provide such training opportunities alongside an expanding community of dedicated professionals. With a focus on inclusive practices and tailored approaches, I host these enriching programs through our platform at www.bempongtalkingtherapy.comwww.bempongtalkingtherapy.com.

Training programs can also cater to the specifics of different cultural groups, like LGBTQ+ individuals, immigrants, or indigenous communities.

Gaining insights into these unique cultural contexts equips participants to understand and address the challenges these communities face, contributing to more culturally conscious care.

In addition, participants may benefit from experiences that foster cultural immersion and offer ongoing supervision. Engaging with experienced professionals in the field can further enhance their grasp of cultural consciousness. In our increasingly interconnected world, this continuous learning and adaptation become vital for anyone keen to improve their understanding and respect for diverse cultural backgrounds. It improves interpersonal relationships, improves interpersonal relationships, and contributes to a more inclusive and empathetic society.

3. **Fostering Inclusive Conversations:**
   Empowering diversity, broadening horizons, and authentic cross-cultural dialogue proves instrumental for professionals striving to deliver culturally conscious care. By intentionally engaging in conversations with individuals of varied backgrounds, these professionals can enrich their understanding of distinct cultural experiences, viewpoints, and healing practices. Such engagement cultivates mutual respect, deepens comprehension, and strengthens the therapeutic alliance. Through a receptive, non-judgmental exchange, professionals can forge safe spaces where clients freely express their cultural identity, navigate cultural stressors, and collaborate in devising effective care plans.

For instance, professionals might organise regular cultural consultation sessions or focus groups, inviting individuals of diverse cultural backgrounds to voice their experiences and perspectives on mental health. These interactions can assist professionals in pinpointing areas of misconception, challenging ingrained biases, and fine-tuning their approaches to better cater to the needs of their culturally diverse clientele.

Culturally Conscious Care in the Workforce: Leading by Example.

Beyond the therapeutic setting, mental health professionals can influence change within the broader workforce and society. They can create transformative shifts in attitudes and practises by championing culturally conscious care practices and promoting diversity, equity, and inclusion.

1. **Advocacy and Policy Initiatives: Driving Systemic Change.**

Mental health professionals can advocate for policies and initiatives that prioritise culturally conscious care and address disparities within the mental health system. By collaborating with policymakers, professional organisations, and community stakeholders, they can influence the development and implementation of policies that promote equitable access to mental health services for all individuals, regardless of their cultural backgrounds. This may involve advocating for increased funding for culturally specific mental health programmes, encouraging diversity in the mental health workforce, and pushing for policy changes that address social determinants of mental health.

2. Mentorship and Education: Empowering the Next Generation.

Mental health professionals have a unique opportunity to mentor and educate the next generation of mental health practitioners. By sharing their knowledge, experiences, and commitment to culturally conscious care, they can inspire and empower future professionals to prioritise cultural consciousness and inclusive practices. Mentoring relationships, workshops, and educational programmes can equip aspiring mental health professionals with the necessary skills and mindset to provide effective and culturally conscious care.

3. Leading by Example: Embracing Diversity and Inclusion.

As leaders in the field, mental health professionals can foster diversity and inclusion within their organisations and professional networks. They can actively recruit and promote professionals from diverse cultural backgrounds, create inclusive policies and practices, and foster a culture of respect and appreciation for cultural differences. By embodying the values of culturally conscious care, they can serve as role models for others in the mental health workforce and drive positive change at both the individual and systemic levels.

Culturally conscious care is not a mere buzzword but a powerful catalyst for transformation in mental health care. It requires mental health professionals to embark on a journey of self-reflection, engage in ongoing learning, and embrace cross-cultural dialogue. By integrating cultural consciousness into their therapeutic practice, advocating for systemic change, and fostering inclusivity within the workforce, mental health professionals can profoundly impact the lives of their clients and the broader community.

Now is the time for mental health professionals to rise to the challenge, take a stand for cultural consciousness, and actively work towards creating a world where everyone receives respectful, inclusive, and genuinely transformative care. By embracing cultural consciousness with passion and dedication, mental health professionals can create a future where mental health care is a beacon of hope, understanding, and healing for all. Let us embark on this journey together and shape a future where cultural consciousness is at the heart of mental health care.

Embracing Cultural Factors in Mental Health: A Personal Journey of Overcoming Racism in Therapy

In mental health, integrating cultural factors is pivotal in providing inclusive and supportive care. Firsthand experiences, like my own, highlight the importance of recognising and addressing racial stereotypes and microaggressions that can inadvertently perpetuate harm within therapeutic settings. By sharing my story, I hope to foster empathy and encourage mental health professionals to actively embrace cultural considerations, thus facilitating a safe and inclusive environment for all individuals seeking support.

My Journey of Seeking Therapy: Like many others, I reached a point where I desperately needed professional support to navigate the challenges I faced. After mustering the courage to seek therapy, I hoped to find solace, understanding, and guidance on my journey towards healing. However, what awaited me in those therapy sessions was an unexpected encounter with racism in the form of stereotypes and microaggressions.

Stereotyping and Microaggressions: A Barrier to Healing During my therapy sessions, I noticed that my experiences as a person of colour were often dismissed or overlooked. My unique cultural background and the challenges I faced due to racial discrimination were rarely acknowledged. Instead, my therapist saw me through a narrow lens shaped by societal stereotypes. Their well-intentioned yet misguided assumptions about my experiences undermined the therapeutic process and hindered my progress.

Microaggressions, often subtle and unintentional, further exacerbated the challenges I encountered. From dismissive comments about the impact of racism on my mental health to insensitive questions about cultural practices, these microaggressions eroded my sense of safety. They hindered my ability to engage in therapy fully. It felt as if the same space meant to provide solace became a reminder of the systemic biases and racial insensitivities I faced daily.

The Transformation through Integrated Cultural Factors: Reflecting upon my experience, I envision a different path—one where the cultural factor is genuinely integrated into the training and practice of mental health professionals like Holly. If cultural considerations had been at the forefront of her practice, my therapy experience could have been radically different.

By acknowledging and understanding the impact of racial stereotypes and microaggressions, Holly could have created a safe and inclusive therapeutic space. She would have recognised the unique challenges I faced due to racial discrimination, validating my experiences rather than dismissing them. Through culturally sensitive assessments, Holly could have delved deeper into the nuances of my cultural background, thus gaining a more comprehensive understanding of my mental health concerns.

Additionally, an integrated approach would have allowed Holly to tailor treatment strategies that addressed the specific hurdles they needed to overcome. By incorporating culturally adapted interventions, such as exploring the effects of intergenerational trauma or discussing the impact of acculturation, therapy could have addressed the root causes of my distress, empowering me to navigate my unique cultural landscape with resilience and strength.

The Power of Culturally Conscious Therapy: If cultural consciousness had been integrated into Holly's training and practice, my therapy journey would have been characterised by support, understanding, and growth. I would have felt seen, heard and understood, knowing that my racial identity and its associated challenges were acknowledged and valued. The therapy seat would have represented a space where I could authentically explore my experiences and work towards healing, free from the weight of racial biases.

My story highlights the transformative potential of embracing cultural consciousness in mental health practice. It serves as a call to action for mental health professionals to recognise the impact of racism, stereotypes, and microaggressions on individuals seeking therapy. By actively integrating cultural considerations, therapists like Holly can create an environment where all clients, regardless of their racial or cultural backgrounds, feel validated, supported, and empowered on their journey to mental well-being.

Our shared experiences navigating the issue of racism in therapy highlight how important it is for mental health professionals to understand and include cultural differences in their work. This step is crucial for breaking down barriers, creating a safe environment for healing, and promoting successful outcomes in therapy. As those seeking help, we all deserve to be seen and understood, including the unique aspects of our cultural identities. Through a solid commitment to understanding and respecting cultural differences, mental health professionals can make a difference in their clients' lives, helping them overcome challenges and find the support they need.

Embracing Cultural Factors in Mental Health: Enhancing Assessment, Diagnosis, and Treatment Planning

In mental health, recognising and incorporating cultural factors into assessment, diagnosis, and treatment planning is vital to providing effective and inclusive care. Cultural consciousness in mental health practice involves understanding how cultural beliefs, values, norms, and experiences shape individuals' mental health concerns. By integrating cultural considerations, mental health professionals can ensure accurate diagnoses, develop tailored treatment plans, and foster meaningful therapeutic relationships. This section explores the significance of cultural consciousness in mental health care. It provides practical strategies, examples, and a case study to illustrate how professionals can effectively integrate cultural consciousness into their practice.

The Significance of Cultural Consciousness: Culture profoundly influences individuals' perceptions, beliefs, and behaviours regarding mental health. It shapes their help-seeking behaviours, views on mental illness, and treatment preferences. Incorporating cultural consciousness into mental health practice acknowledges the diversity of human experiences, promotes cultural humility, and improves therapeutic outcomes.

Cultural Consciousness in Assessment:

- **Language and Communication**: Language issues can cause problems with accurate assessments. For instance, a client might need to be more fluent in the language the therapy is provided, which can lead to misunderstandings or an inability to express complex emotions fully. Treatment is provided, which can lead to misunderstandings or a failure to express complicated feelings fully. Therefore, mental health professionals should give language interpreters or use culturally sensitive assessment tools that cater to different linguistic backgrounds.

An example would be a questionnaire translated and culturally adapted into the client's mother tongue. In addition, understanding cultural communication patterns can also enhance assessments. For instance, in some cultures, direct eye contact might be considered redirect eye contact might be considered rude, while in others, it could indicate engagement. Recognising these non-verbal cues and idiomatic expressions like local phrases or proverbs can enrich the therapeutic dialogue and make assessments more accurate and meaningful.

b) Beliefs and Values: A person's cultural beliefs and values significantly impact how they perceive mental health, their attitude towards getting help, and what they expect from treatment.

For instance, in some cultures, mental health issues might be attributed to spiritual or supernatural causes, affecting their willingness to seek conventional mental health treatment. In other cultures, seeking help for mental health issues might be seen as a sign of weakness or may carry a stigma, deterring individuals from reaching out.

It's crucial for professionals to actively explore and recognise these cultural factors to understand where their clients are coming from fully. By doing this, they can adjust their approach to assessment. For example, a practitioner may incorporate religious or spiritual elements into therapy if that aligns with the client's beliefs and would incorporate religious or spiritual aspects into treatment if that aligns with the client's beliefs and makes them more comfortable with the process.

Cultural Factors in Diagnosis:

a) Cultural Formulation Interview (CFI): The CFI, developed by the American Psychiatric Association, is a valuable tool for systematically evaluating an individual's cultural context. It assists in identifying cultural influences on symptom presentation, distress, and functioning, leading to more accurate diagnoses.

b) Diverse Symptom Expression: Mental health symptoms can manifest differently across cultures. For example, certain cultures may emphasise physical somatic symptoms over psychological distress, which can lead to underdiagnosis or misdiagnosis. Professionals can avoid pathologising regular cultural expressions and ensure accurate diagnoses by attuning to these cultural variations.

Cultural Factors in Treatment Planning:

a) Culturally Adapted Interventions: Tailoring interventions to align with cultural beliefs, practises, and values enhance treatment outcomes. For instance, incorporating traditional healing practices, spirituality or involving extended family members in therapy can be crucial in particular cultural contexts.

b) Lifestyle Determinants: Cultural factors influence an individual's lifestyle determinants, such as diet, exercise, and social support systems, which impact mental health. Professionals should consider these cultural lifestyle determinants when developing treatment plans to address clients ' needs and preferences.

Less Obvious Examples:

a) Historical and Intergenerational Trauma: Historical events, such as colonisation, slavery, or genocide, can have long-lasting effects on individuals and communities. Understanding the cultural impact of such traumas is essential for mental health professionals to provide sensitive care and support healing.

b) Acculturation and Immigration Stress: Immigrants and individuals undergoing the acculturation process often face unique stressors, such as language barriers, discrimination, and identity conflicts. By acknowledging these challenges and considering the cultural adjustment process, professionals can tailor treatment approaches to address their clients ' needs.

Case Study: Culturally Conscious Approach in Practice.

Consider the following example of a mental health practitioner working with a client of West African heritage named Yaa. Yaa exhibits symptoms consistent with anxiety and a tendency towards perfectionism. However, it's essential to appreciate that her cultural roots significantly influence these symptoms' presentation.

Coming from a West African background, Yaa is likely subject to a cultural experience that places considerable emphasis on academic excellence and fulfilling family expectations. This cultural context might contribute to her feelings of anxiety and her drive to perfectionism, both of which are understandable responses to the high expectations she feels compelled to meet.

Recognising these cultural influences, mental health practitioner integrates these considerations into their assessment and subsequent treatment plan. They employ standard cognitive-behavioural therapy techniques to address Yaa's anxiety and perfectionistic tendencies. They also use traditional cognitive-behavioural therapy techniques to manage Yaa's anxiety and perfectionistic tendencies and weave strategies that acknowledge her cultural pressures.

For example, the practitioner might work with Yaa on developing stress management strategies that respect her cultural values. They might suggest mindfulness techniques that echo traditional West African meditation practices, or they may facilitate discussions around setting healthy boundaries with family members.

Furthermore, their sessions become a platform for Yaa to discuss the cultural expectations she experiences openly. By providing a safe space to voice these cultural pressures, the professional empowers Yaa to navigate her unique struggles, acknowledging her cultural reality while enabling her to address her mental health needs.

By integrating this culturally conscious approach, the mental health professional develops a personalised treatment plan that fully appreciates Yaa's cultural context, ultimately fostering a more impactful therapeutic relationship.

Integrating cultural factors into mental health assessment, diagnosis, and treatment planning is crucial for providing effective and inclusive care. By recognising the impact of culture on individuals' mental health experiences and tailoring interventions accordingly, professionals can foster trust, enhance treatment outcomes, and promote overall well-being. Embracing cultural factors is an ongoing process that requires cultural humility, self-reflection, and a commitment to continuous learning. By actively engaging in culturally conscious practises mental health professionals contribute to a more equitable and accessible mental health care system.

Intersecting Identities: Navigating My Journey as a Black, Gay, and Dyslexic Individual

My journey as a Black, gay, and dyslexic individual has been a transformative exploration of the intersecting identities that constitute my essence. The unique challenges I've encountered along this path, exacerbated by the potent effects of intersectional marginalisation, have profoundly shaped my mental well-being. Yet, through the valuable tools of therapy, self-discovery, and resilience, I've been able to work through these adversities, find self-acceptance, and have worked through these adversities, found self-acceptance, and pave a path marked by understanding and empathy.

Understanding Multiple Identities:

Being a Black, gay, and dyslexic man involved coming to terms with multiple dimensions of my identity. In this early phase of my journey, I faced the harsh reality of intersectional marginalisation. The societal pressures to conform pushed me into pockets of limited acceptance, igniting a struggle with my self-perception and sense of worth.

Confronting Intersectional Marginalization:

As I delved deeper into my journey, the nuanced complexities of intersectional marginalisation became more apparent. This layered oppression introduced me to a labyrinth of emotional and psychological hurdles. Experiences of rejection and exclusion from loved ones amplified these challenges, leaving lasting emotional scars and highlighting the pressing need for supportive and fair systems. However, it's essential to remember that if you've experienced rejection due to intersecting identities, you're not alone. We can collaboratively nurture a society that acknowledges and values diversity and fosters environments where everyone feels seen, heard, and accepted.

Struggling Towards Self-Acceptance:

The world often imposes narrow societal roles and expectations, making the journey towards self-acceptance arduous. Negative messages of worthlessness, coupled with rejection and exclusion, feelings of worthlessness and sacrifice, and exclusion worsened the struggle. Recognising the need for change, I realised the importance of support from mental health professionals, workplaces, and societies. We have the collective power to challenge stereotypes, provide culturally conscious care, and foster inclusive environments, cultivating a culture that appreciates uniqueness and intersectionality.

Finding Refuge in Culturally Conscious Therapy:

Culturally Conscious Therapy was a sanctuary in my journey, facilitating healing and self-discovery. In this haven, I could confront the compounding effects of intersectional marginalisation and navigate the deep-seated scars of discrimination, rejection and exclusion. Culturally Conscious Therapy empowered me to question societal narratives, dismantle internalised oppression, and nurture self-compassion – tools that have been instrumental in building resilience and navigating the complexities of my identities.

Revelation and Transformation:

A critical juncture in my journey came when I realised that my intersecting identities are not burdens but sources of strength. I found the courage to reject societal expectations and embrace my true self, marking a crucial step towards self-acceptance. This transformative phase taught me to extend compassion towards myself and others, accept the diverse nature of human existence, and exercise patience when dealing with intersectional identities.

Growth and Discovery:

The culmination of my journey as a Black, gay, and dyslexic man has been marked by profound growth, resilience, and self-discovery. I've weathered the impacts of intersectional marginalisation, amplified by rejection and exclusion from loved ones. These experiences have significantly influenced my mental health. However, with therapy, self-reflection, and resilience, I've embarked on a journey of self-acceptance and compassion. By sharing my story, I hope to provide understanding and inspiration to others navigating similar paths, contributing to a more inclusive and empathetic society.

Cultivating Cultural Consciousness and Embracing Intersectionality in Therapy: Enhancing Mental Health Professionals' Awareness

In the dynamic field of mental health, it is essential for professionals to continuously strive for cultural consciousness and a deep understanding of intersectionality. By recognising clients' diverse cultural backgrounds, identities, and experiences, mental health professionals can supply more inclusive and effective therapy. This section explores how mental health professionals can enhance their cultural consciousness and awareness of intersectionality, fostering a therapeutic environment that is sensitive, respectful, and empowering.

Understanding Cultural Consciousness: Cultural consciousness in therapy refers to the ability of mental health professionals to work with individuals from diverse cultural backgrounds. It entails developing knowledge, attitudes, and skills that allow therapists to navigate the complexities of culture and its influence on mental health. Mental health professionals must engage in ongoing self-reflection, education, and active learning to enhance cultural consciousness.

- **Self-Reflection:** Recognising Personal Biases
The first step in cultivating cultural consciousness is for mental health professionals to self-reflect and acknowledge their biases. Personal beliefs, values, and experiences shape our perspectives, and awareness of these influences is crucial to supplying unbiased and culturally conscious care. By examining their assumptions and prejudices, therapists can better understand how these might affect their therapeutic relationships and tailor their approach accordingly.

- **Education and Training:** Mental health professionals should actively seek education and training opportunities focusing on cultural consciousness. This may involve attending workshops, conferences, or seminars on topics such as cultural diversity, cultural humility, and cultural sensitivity. These initiatives supply valuable insights into diverse cultural groups' experiences, histories, and unique challenges.

- **Developing Knowledge and Understanding:** To enhance cultural competence, mental health professionals must familiarise themselves with the cultural norms, values, and traditions of their communities. This can be achieved through reading literature, conversing with individuals from diverse backgrounds, and seeking guidance from cultural consultants or experts. By expanding their knowledge base, therapists can better understand and confirm their clients' experiences while avoiding stereotyping or generalisations.

- **Active Listening and Empathy:** An integral aspect of cultural consciousness is listening actively and empathising with clients. Mental health professionals should create a safe space for clients to express their thoughts, emotions, and cultural perspectives without fear of judgment or discrimination. By listening attentively and showing empathy, therapists can validate clients' experiences and foster a therapeutic alliance built on trust.

Addressing Intersectionality in Therapy:

Intersectionality recognises that individuals have multiple social identities that intersect and interact, shaping their experiences and challenges. Mental health professionals must know these intersections and understand how they affect their clients' lives. Here are some strategies for enhancing awareness of intersectionality in therapy:

1. **Recognising Privilege and Power Dynamics:** Therapists must acknowledge their privilege and power dynamics within the therapeutic relationship. This requires understanding how societal structures and systems may affect clients differently based on their intersecting identities. Owning these

power dynamics allows mental health professionals to create a more egalitarian and empowering therapeutic environment.

2. **Tailoring Treatment Approaches:** Through tailored treatment approaches, effective therapy acknowledges and addresses clients' unique experiences and needs. By considering the intersectional identities of their clients, mental health professionals can adapt therapeutic techniques to suit their circumstances better. For example, a therapist collaborating with a queer person of colour may need to explore the impact of racism, homophobia, and cultural expectations on their mental health.

3. **Collaborative Approach**: Inclusive therapy involves collective decision-making between therapists and clients. Mental health professionals should actively involve clients in treatment planning, allowing them to express their needs, goals, and preferences. This collaborative approach ensures that therapy considers clients' intersecting identities and lived experiences, leading to more meaningful and relevant interventions.

Case Study: Harnessing Intersectional Awareness in Therapy - Anansi's Journey

Anansi, a young African British man, sought therapy to address his battles with anxiety and depression. His prior experience with treatment felt dissatisfying, as he sensed his cultural background was consistently sidelined. This oversight led to a disconnect and stalled progress in his treatment. However, when he started therapy sessions with me, an advocate of intersectionality and cultural consciousness, the dynamics began to change significantly.

Understanding the unique challenges Anansi faced as a Black man was pivotal. I acknowledged the complex realities of his experience, such as racial microaggressions and intergenerational trauma. Viewing his situation through an intersectional lens, I aimed to incorporate cultural factors into the treatment plan, utilising techniques such as narrative therapy and exploring the impact of racial identity on Anansi's mental well-being.

As a result of this holistic, culturally aware approach, Anansi felt validated and understood. He felt empowered to address his mental health concerns within the broader context of his cultural identity. This approach brought a sense of relevancy and authenticity to his therapeutic journey, opening avenues for improved mental health outcomes.

In an increasingly diverse world, mental health professionals must strive to enhance their cultural consciousness and awareness of intersectionality. Therapists can create an inclusive and empowering therapeutic environment by fostering a deeper understanding of cultural factors, recognising privilege, and acknowledging the unique challenges faced by individuals with intersecting identities. Through ongoing self-reflection, education, and active listening, mental health professionals can effectively integrate cultural factors into assessment, diagnosis, and treatment planning, improving therapeutic outcomes for their clients.

Embracing Diversity: Collaborative and Inclusive Mental Health Care for Intersectional Marginalised Identities

In today's diverse society, mental health professionals are crucial in providing inclusive and effective care for individuals with intersectional marginalised identities. The UK is a multicultural nation comprising various ethnicities, religions, genders, sexual orientations, and abilities. However, with diversity come unique challenges that impact mental health and well-being. This section explores the importance of collaborative and inclusive mental health care while highlighting individuals' distinctive challenges with intersectional marginalised identities. By delving into different examples and contexts, we can shed light on the complexities of mental health experiences and the necessity of a culturally conscious approach.

Understanding Intersectionality: The concept of intersectionality resonates strongly within the UK, given its diverse population and history of multiculturalism. Mental health professionals must grasp the nuances of intersectionality and acknowledge how various intersecting identities shape an individual's mental health experiences. For instance, a Black lesbian woman with a disability in the UK may face discrimination, misogyny, homophobia, racism, and ableism, all of which impact her mental well-being. By recognising intersectionality, mental health professionals can adapt their assessments, diagnoses, and treatment plans to meet the specific needs of individuals in the UK.

Navigating Intersectionality in Mental Health: Tackling the Complex Challenges of Highly Marginalized Intersecting Identities

Effectively addressing mental health challenges necessitates a thorough understanding of intersectionality, acknowledging the overlapping facets of an individual's identity that shape their life experiences. People with highly marginalised intersecting identities frequently encounter intensified systemic discrimination, social exclusion, and internalised oppression, leading to distinct and multifaceted mental health concerns.

Let's delve into some examples of the most marginalised intersecting identities to illustrate this complexity:

1. **Transgender Women of Colour:** Individuals in this group face heightened stigmatisation due to the intersection of their race and gender identity. Experiencing racism and transphobia simultaneously

often leads to increased violence, discrimination, and consequent mental health issues, alongside barriers to accessing quality healthcare services.

2. **Disabled Immigrants from Ethnic Minority Groups: For** any immigrant, adapting to a new cultural environment can be challenging adjusting to a new cultural environment can be challenging. Still, this challenge is significantly amplified for those from ethnic minority backgrounds with disabilities. These individuals face exacerbated isolation and mental distress due to language barriers, the absence of culturally conscious support services, and the intersecting prejudices of xenophobia and ableism.

3. **Elderly LGBTQ+ Individuals with Disabilities: The** convergence of ageism, homophobia or transphobia, and ableism places elderly LGBTQ+ individuals with disabilities at a distinct disadvantage. They may struggle with discrimination within both age-related and LGBTQ+ services. Their unique needs often go unaddressed due to a lack of understanding and awareness.

4. **LGBTQ+ Individuals from Ethnic and Religious Minority Groups**: These individuals may experience dissonance between their sexual orientation or gender identity and their cultural or religious beliefs, leading to conflicts with family and community. The co-existence of homophobia, racism, and religious intolerance can result in heightened mental health challenges such as anxiety and depression.

5. **Black Women with Neurodiverse Conditions and Lower Socioeconomic Status:** This group encounters the intersection of racial, gender,

socioeconomic, and neurodivergent bias. Societal stereotypes, economic disparities, and expectations can contribute to elevated stress levels and feelings of isolation. Their unique needs may often be overlooked due to prevailing biases and systemic inequities.

6. **Indigenous LGBTQ+ Individuals:** The intersection of indigenous identity and LGBTQ+ identity presents unique challenges. These individuals often face societal prejudices based on their ethnic background and sexual orientation or gender identity, resulting in amplified mental distress and potential barriers to accessing culturally sensitive mental health services.

By understanding these intersecting identities, mental health professionals are better equipped to develop inclusive, personalised, and equitable mental health interventions. This intersectionality-aware approach enables the recognition of unique challenges faced by highly marginalised individuals, promoting a more holistic approach to mental health care and fostering a higher probability of positive treatment outcomes.

Promoting Cultural Consciousness in Global Mental Health Care:

Emphasising the importance of cultural consciousness within global mental health care is paramount. Mental health professionals worldwide are responsible for actively understanding each individual's diverse artistic practices, values, and beliefs. They must recognise the distinct challenges marginalised communities encounter due to systemic structures and societal norms in various corners of the globe.

Integrating Cultural Consciousness into Care: A conscious integration of cultural consciousness into their professional practice is a powerful tool that mental health professionals can utilise. Doing so can foster a secure and affirming environment where clients feel genuinely seen and acknowledged. This approach extends beyond mere tolerance, inviting professionals to continually reflect on their potential biases, challenge stereotypes, and commit to ongoing learning to uphold an exemplary standard of culturally conscious care.

The Power of Collaboration and Trust: Collaboration and trust-building are critical in establishing successful therapeutic relationships. Professionals empower clients to voice their unique perspectives, ambitions, and personal preferences by nurturing a collaborative rapport with individuals from diverse backgrounds. Professionals enable clients to express their amazing views, dreams, and personal preferences by fostering a collective camaraderie with individuals from diverse backgrounds. This connection cultivates a space of trust, enabling clients to feel esteemed and validated. Such a robust therapeutic alliance allows mental health professionals to comprehensively understand clients' intersectional experiences, fine-tuning interventions to each individual's needs.

Advancing Intersectionality-Informed Interventions on a Global Scale:

There is an urgent need for mental health professionals globally to devise and deploy interventions specifically designed to meet the needs of individuals with intersecting marginalised identities.

3 Practical steps:

1. Facilitating support groups or community networks that unite individuals with similar intersectional identities, offering a haven for shared experiences and mutual understanding.

2. Orchestrating targeted workshops or training sessions to equip professionals with the tools to deepen their understanding of cultural consciousness and intersectionality.

3. Forging partnerships with community organisations and advocates to co-create culturally responsive resources and interventions tailored to honour diverse identities.

Mental health professionals worldwide need to champion diversity and adopt inclusive; collaborative care approaches when working with individuals with intersecting marginalised identities. Recognising these individuals' unique mental health challenges and nurturing cultural consciousness is vital for devising more effective and empowering interventions. By cultivating a therapeutic space that respects and values diverse identities, mental health professionals can significantly enhance mental well-being globally, steering us towards a more inclusive and equitable society.

There is a dire need for mental health professionals to adopt intersectionality-informed approaches in their practice. By facilitating support networks, providing intersectionality-focused training, and creating culturally responsive resources, we can provide more effective care to individuals with intersecting marginalised identities. This requires a worldwide commitment to champion diversity, inclusivity, and collaboration in mental health care. We can significantly enhance global mental well-being by acknowledging these individuals' unique mental health challenges and cultivating an environment that respects and values diverse identities. This is a vital step towards a more inclusive and equitable society.

Chapter 3 Key Points:

1. **Unleashing the Power of Cultural Consciousness**: Mental health care providers must recognise the diversity of individuals' experiences, identities, and cultural backgrounds to provide tailored and effective therapy. Culturally conscious care allows mental health professionals to understand their client's unique needs, fostering inclusivity and positive change.

2. **Understanding Cultural Consciousness**: Cultural consciousness involves deeply understanding and respecting diverse cultures, beliefs, and values. It requires professionals to recognise how societal, historical, and

systemic factors influence mental health, equipping them with the tools to provide culturally conscious care.

3. **Self-Reflection and Awareness**: The first step towards providing culturally conscious care involves self-reflection and increased awareness of one's biases, assumptions, and cultural perspectives.

4. **Culturally Conscious Care in the Workforce**: Mental health professionals can influence change within the broader workforce and society by promoting culturally conscious care practices and advocating for diversity, equity, and inclusion.

5. **Advocacy and Policy Initiatives**: Professionals can collaborate with policymakers and community stakeholders to advocate for policies prioritising culturally conscious care and addressing disparities in the mental health system.

6. **Personal Journey of Overcoming Racism in Therapy**: The author's experience of racism in therapy highlights the importance of recognising racial stereotypes and microaggressions that can inadvertently perpetuate harm within therapeutic settings.

7. **Cultural Factors in Mental Health Assessment, Diagnosis, and Treatment Planning**: Recognising and incorporating cultural factors into mental health practice is vital for accurate diagnoses, tailored treatment

plans, and meaningful therapeutic relationships.

8. **The Significance of Cultural Consciousness**: Culture profoundly influences individuals' perceptions, beliefs, and behaviours regarding mental health. Incorporating cultural consciousness into mental health practice acknowledges this diversity, promotes cultural humility, and improves therapeutic outcomes.

9. **Intersecting Identities**: The author shares their experience as a Black, gay, and dyslexic individual to highlight the importance of understanding intersectionality in mental health care. The unique challenges faced due to intersectional marginalisation can significantly impact mental health.

10. **Cultivating Cultural Consciousness and Embracing Intersectionality in Therapy**: Mental health professionals can enhance their cultural consciousness and understanding of intersectionality to provide more inclusive and effective therapy.

11. **Navigating Intersectionality in Mental Health**: Recognising the complexities of intersectionality is crucial for addressing the unique mental health challenges faced by people with highly marginalised intersecting identities.

12. **Advancing Intersectionality-Informed Interventions on a Global Scale**: Mental

health professionals globally need to create interventions specifically designed to meet the needs of individuals with intersecting marginalised identities. This may involve facilitating support groups, orchestrating targeted training sessions, and partnering with community organisations to create culturally responsive resources.

Our role in promoting antiracism is crucial. Embrace chosen family and allyship. Challenge oppressive systems. Create an inclusive society. Let us embark on the Hero's Journey of allyship, dismantling discrimination and embracing all.

Jarell Bempong

Chapter 4

Antiracism and Allyship: Mental Health Professionals and Individuals as Agents of Change

Embracing Chosen Family: Antiracism and Allyship in the Journey of Resilience

Within the intricate tapestry of my journey as a Black, gay, dyslexic individual in a society deeply rooted in white supremacy, patriarchy, and religious dogmas, the search for allies took on a profound significance. The rejection, humiliation, hurt, abuse, ridicule, and constant sense of being overlooked, unheard, unseen, unaccepted, and misunderstood pushed me to seek solace beyond traditional notions of family. In this exploration, I discovered my chosen family's power and resilience.

As I longed for acceptance and understanding within my biological family, the pain of their inability to fully embrace and affirm my identity was deeply felt. The yearning for connection and unconditional love, however, did not fade. In my quest, I found solace and belonging in the arms of my chosen family. These are the individuals who, through shared experiences and empathetic hearts, embraced me for who I am without judgment or conditions. They saw the scars inflicted by a society that perpetuated injustice and inequality, and they stood beside me as pillars of unwavering support.

The chosen family represents a transformative bond that transcends blood ties. It is a web of relationships forged through shared struggles, understanding, and determined acceptance. In the darkest moments, when rejection and pain seemed insurmountable, the chosen family became the refuge, offering unconditional love, compassion, and a listening ear. They became the mirrors that reflected my true worth and the sounding boards for my dreams and aspirations. Together, we created a space where authenticity thrived, where our shared journeys intertwined to form a tapestry of resilience and strength.

The significance of the chosen family lies in the power of collective healing. Through their presence, I discovered that the wounds inflicted by rejection, humiliation, and abuse could be transformed into spaces of growth and empowerment. We held open for one another's pain, weaving threads of love, support, and understanding into our shared existence. In embracing my chosen family, I learned to redefine notions of kinship and create a sense of belonging rooted in compassion and acceptance.

However, the journey of finding my chosen family was challenging. It required a willingness to relinquish societal expectations and redefine what familial bonds mean to me. It demanded courage to detach from toxic relationships and release the pain caused by those unable or unwilling to see my worth. It was a process of shedding the layers of hurt and rebuilding a support system that celebrated my identity and championed my growth.

To those who have experienced rejection, humiliation, pain, abuse, ridicule, overlooked, unheard, unseen, unaccepted, and misunderstood, chosen family offers a lifeline. It is a testament to the human capacity for resilience and the power of love to heal deep wounds. It reminds us that we are not defined by the limitations imposed upon us by others but rather by the strength and compassion we find within ourselves and those who choose to stand by our side.

As I continue my journey, I hold my chosen family and the concept of allies close to my heart. They are the beacons of light guiding me through the darkness, reminding me that I am not alone in my struggles. They inspire me to be an ally to others, extending a hand of support and understanding to those who have experienced similar pain and longing for acceptance. Together, we navigate the complexities of a world that often fails to recognise our worth. We find solace, empowerment, and hope in the transformative power of chosen family and the unwavering bonds of allyship.

In the fight against systemic racism, oppression, and discrimination, antiracism and allyship become crucial pillars of change. Mental health professionals and individuals alike have the power to dismantle the harmful narratives and structures that perpetuate inequality and injustice. By recognising the importance of chosen family, we understand the significance of creating safe spaces where all individuals, regardless of their backgrounds, can find acceptance, love, and support.

Through the lens of antiracism, we actively challenge the systems that perpetuate white supremacy and work towards creating an inclusive and equitable society. We educate ourselves and others, confront our biases, and actively seek to dismantle oppressive structures. As allies, we use our voices, platforms, and resources to amplify marginalised voices, advocate for their rights, and create spaces for their stories to be heard and valued.

The journey towards antiracism and allyship has its challenges. It requires self-reflection, humility, and a commitment to continuous learning and growth. It demands that we confront our privilege and use it to uplift others. But in doing so, we contribute to the collective resilience and empowerment of those who have been rejected, humiliated, hurt, abused, ridiculed, overlooked, unheard, unseen, unaccepted, and misunderstood.

Embracing chosen family and committing to antiracism and allyship is a transformative act of love and solidarity. It acknowledges the interconnectedness of our struggles and our power to create change. Together, we can forge a path towards a more just and inclusive society where everyone, regardless of their identities, can thrive, be celebrated, and find solace in embracing a chosen family that stands firmly against oppression and inequality.

The Power of Allyship: Challenging Inequality and Amplifying Marginalised Voices

In our collective pursuit of equality and justice, it is crucial to recognise the immense power of allyship. Allies, particularly those belonging to the majority or dominant groups, are uniquely positioned to challenge inequality and uplift the voices of marginalised communities. This chapter explores the responsibilities of allies and the transformative impact they can have on dismantling systemic discrimination. Supporters can contribute to a more inclusive and just society by leveraging their privileges and advocating for equity.

Understanding Allyship: Allyship is not merely an identity but a verb, an ongoing commitment to dismantling oppressive systems. It involves individuals who belong to privileged groups actively using their positions to challenge discrimination, amplify marginalised voices, and advocate for meaningful change. True allyship requires self-reflection, education, and a willingness to confront biases and blind spots.

The Power of Privilege: Privilege refers to the inherent advantages and benefits that individuals enjoy based on their social identities. It can manifest in various forms, such as racial, gender, or socioeconomic privilege. Acknowledging one's privilege is the first step towards becoming an effective ally. Recognising that privilege is not a personal failing, but rather a systemic advantage is essential to understanding the role one can play in dismantling inequality.

The Responsibility of Allies: If an individual belongs to the majority or dominant group in society, enjoys the default privileges associated with that group, yet remains passive in the face of discrimination, they inadvertently perpetuate inequality. Allies are morally obligated to actively challenge injustice and use their voices of privilege to uplift marginalised voices. It is not enough to be a silent observer; allies must actively engage in the fight against systemic discrimination.

1. **Amplifying Marginalised Voices:** One of the most significant roles of allies is amplifying the voices of marginalised communities. By actively listening, learning, and centring the experiences and perspectives of those who face systemic barriers, allies can bring attention to issues that often go unnoticed or ignored. This involves advocating for marginalised voices to be heard in spaces where decisions are made, whether in the workplace, education, politics, or community organisations.

2. **Using Privilege for Systemic Change:** Allies must leverage their privileges to advocate for equitable policies, practises, and systemic changes. This requires acting, engaging in uncomfortable conversations, and challenging discriminatory practices wherever they may exist. It also involves examining one's biases and unlearning harmful stereotypes, as true allyship begins with personal growth and transformation.

The Hero's Journey of Allyship: Learning from Joseph Campbell's Narrative Archetype

Embodying the ideals of an ally in today's diverse and rapidly evolving societies is akin to undertaking a Hero's Journey, a concept brought to light by renowned scholar and mythologist Joseph Campbell. His concept of the Hero's Journey, a narrative pattern common to stories worldwide, offers a robust framework for understanding the path towards becoming an effective ally.

Joseph Campbell's Contribution: Campbell's seminal work, The Hero with a Thousand Faces, introduced the concept of the Hero's Journey or the monomyth. His idea suggests that all mythic narratives are variations of a single great story — a pattern that profoundly resonates with the human experience. This journey involves stages such as the call to adventure, the meeting with a mentor, facing and overcoming trials, and the return with newfound wisdom. In the context of allyship, this concept underscores the iterative and transformative process of self-discovery, learning, and active advocacy.

The Hero's Journey of Allyship: A Path Towards Advocacy and Inclusion

1. **The Call to Adventure:** Embarking on the allyship journey starts with the "call to adventure," a desire to deepen one's understanding of marginalised communities. This stage involves active learning about the historical context of oppression, systemic barriers, and the lived experiences of marginalised groups. The journey is continuous and challenging, demanding engagement with diverse perspectives and resources.

2. **Meeting the Mentor and Gaining Allies:** As in Campbell's monomyth, the ally's journey also benefits from mentors — individuals,

communities, or resources that provide knowledge and guidance. Simultaneously, the aspiring ally begins to recognise personal biases and privilege, an essential step towards self-awareness and growth.

3. **Trials, Tests and the Ordeal**: The true test of an ally comes in the form of active advocacy. Using one's privilege to confront and challenge discriminatory practices represents the ordeal, the decisive ordeal or crisis in one's journey. Allies are called to speak out against injustice in personal and broader social contexts.

4. **The Reward and The Return:** The ally amplifies marginalised voices, sharing their stories and creating platforms for their narratives — the reward. This process transforms the ally and the communities they advocate for, resulting in a return to society with a renewed sense of responsibility and a commitment to ongoing allyship.

Campbell's Hero's Journey provides a compelling metaphor for the allyship journey. It is not a linear process but a cyclical journey of continuous learning, action, and growth. Embracing this journey's inherent challenges and rewards allows allies to progress from silent observers to active agents of change, contributing to a more inclusive, equitable, and just society.

The Power of Amplifying Marginalised Voices: Historical Examples of Allyship

Throughout history, oppressed communities have faced numerous struggles and fought for their rights and freedom. However, it is crucial to acknowledge that actual progress and change only occurred when members of the majority groups amplified the voices of the marginalised, becoming allies in their fight for equality. This section explores historical examples where allyship was pivotal in advancing oppressed communities' rights.

The Civil Rights Movement

The Civil Rights Movement in the United States during the 1950s and 1960s was a turning point in the fight against racial segregation and discrimination. While African Americans led the justice charge, the movement gained significant momentum when white allies recognised the injustice and joined the cause. People like Rosa Parks, a Black woman who refused to give up her bus seat, inspired countless Black and white individuals to unite and demand change. White activists like Viola Liuzzo and James Reeb sacrificed their lives while participating in the movement, collaborating with their black counterparts like Martin Luther King Jr., Malcolm X, and Ella Baker. Together, they organised protests, advocated for policy reforms, and amplified the voices of the marginalised. Their collective efforts helped dismantle legal segregation and pave the way for greater racial equality.

Gay Rights Movement

The struggle for LGBTQ+ rights has seen remarkable progress in recent decades, partly thanks to allyship. Allies from all social classes have played crucial roles in challenging societal norms, advocating for equal rights, and creating safe spaces for LGBTQ+ individuals. The Stonewall Riots 1969, sparked by trans women of colour, led to a widespread LGBTQ+ rights movement. Over time, allies within the heterosexual and cisgender communities recognised the injustices faced by their LGBTQ+ friends, family members, and colleagues. They marched alongside them in pride parades, supported legislative changes, and stood up against discrimination. The fight for marriage equality, as seen in landmark cases like Obergefell v. Hodges, highlighted the strength of allyship in dismantling discriminatory laws.

Apartheid in South Africa

Apartheid was a system of racial segregation and discrimination enforced by the South African government from 1948 to 1994. The fight against apartheid saw widespread international allyship and solidarity. Organisations like the African National Congress (ANC) led the resistance within South Africa, but the global support and pressure contributed to its eventual downfall. People worldwide rallied against apartheid, participating in boycotts, divestments, and protests. Musicians and activists like Bob Marley, Peter Gabriel, and Steven Van Zandt used their platforms to raise awareness and promote unity. Their alliance helped expose the injustices of apartheid and applied pressure on governments and institutions to take a stand against racial segregation.

Suffragettes and Women's Rights

The suffragette movement, which fought for women's right to vote, is another testament to the power of allyship. Women faced widespread disenfranchisement and discrimination in the late 19th and early 20th centuries. However, the movement gained significant momentum when male allies recognised the inherent injustice and supported women's suffrage. Men like Frederick Douglass, a prominent abolitionist, championed women's rights alongside their fight against slavery. Their allyship helped advance the cause, leading to the eventual ratification of the 19th Amendment in the United States, which granted women the right to vote.

George Floyd and the Global Alliance

The tragic murder of George Floyd in 2020 sparked a global movement against racial injustice and police brutality. It was a stark reminder of the urgent need for allies to stand in solidarity with marginalised communities. The Black Lives Matter movement gained widespread support as people from diverse backgrounds, including many from the majority white community, recognised the systemic racism faced by Black individuals. They took to the streets, engaged in complex conversations, and actively challenged the status quo. This alliance helped shed light on the ongoing racial disparities and generated momentum for substantial change in law enforcement practices and systemic racism.

History has shown us that only oppressed groups have achieved their rights and freedom by amplifying their voices with allies from the majority or dominant groups. From the Civil Rights Movement to the fight for LGBTQ+ rights and women's suffrage, allyship has been pivotal in driving social progress. The recent events surrounding George Floyd's death and the resulting alliance demonstrate the ongoing importance of amplifying marginalised voices and actively working towards a more just and inclusive society. As we move forward, let us be inspired by these historical examples and commit ourselves to become allies, using our privileges and voices to challenge discrimination, dismantle systemic barriers, and create lasting change for all.

Activating Change: How Mental Health Professionals Can Advocate for Marginalised Communities

Building Bempong Talking Therapy: A Journey of Cultural Consciousness and Healing

As the founder of Bempong Talking Therapy Ltd., I've authored this book, which encapsulates the journey to establishing our transformative centre. This centre, dedicated to mental health and wellbeing, is deeply committed to culturally conscious care, focusing on Black individuals and other cultural minorities. Bempong Talking Therapy Ltd. stands as a testament to the empathy, compassion, and understanding honed from both personal and collective challenges faced is a testament to the empathy, compassion, and understanding filed from both individual and collective challenges. Our journey and the lessons I've learned are interwoven in the fabric of the centre, contributing to its mission and philosophy.

Origins of Bempong Talking Therapy Ltd:

The journey of establishing Bempong Talking Therapy Ltd. was a complex idea. It was an earnest response to the stark realities of systemic barriers, misconceptions, and lack of representation in conventional therapy settings. The absence of a safe space for healing and empowerment for Black individuals was an obstacle and inspiration in creating the centre.

Cultural Consciousness in Therapy:

Bempong Talking Therapy Ltd. is a testament to the importance of cultural consciousness in therapy. The unique mental health challenges facing the Black community, often shaped by historical oppression, systemic racism, and intergenerational trauma, informed my approach. Embracing and incorporating cultural factors into our therapeutic methods has been fundamental in creating a healing environment that respects and validates the diversity of my client's experiences.

Inclusivity and Empowerment:

I am steadfast in creating a therapy centre where individuals of every cultural identity can feel seen, heard, and understood. Through a lens of empathy and understanding, I have sought to establish an environment where clients can express themselves without fear of judgment or misunderstanding.

Addressing Intersectionality:

Recognising intersectionality is not an afterthought at Bempong Talking Therapy but a core principle. I understand the complex web of identities, encompassing race, gender, sexuality, ability, and socioeconomic status, that our clients navigate. By acknowledging this reality, I've created a space where clients can explore and address the unique mental health challenges presented by their diverse identities.

Resilience and Transformation:

The transformative journeys of my clients have been a wellspring of inspiration and humility. Celebrating their resilience, courage, and growth is crucial to my practice. I aspire to empower clients to reclaim their narratives and embrace their authentic selves through culturally conscious care. My ultimate goal is to equip individuals with the tools and support they need to thrive.

Advocacy and Collaboration:

My work is not confined to individual therapy sessions. We are actively involved in advocacy initiatives and build partnerships with community organisations, striving for systemic change and increased access to mental health resources for marginalised communities.

The Journey Continues:

The commitment to Bempong Talking Therapy is a commitment to growth and evolution. The goal is to expand our services, engage in professional development, and nurture a supportive environment for our therapists, enhancing their cultural consciousness and ensuring we stay at the forefront of mental health care for Black and other cultural minority individuals.

Bempong Talking Therapy's growth has been a labour of love. The Centre has shown the transformative power of culturally conscious care. I invite mental health professionals and aspiring therapists to join me on this journey of cultural consciousness and inclusivity. Together, we can bring about lasting change and build a world where everyone has the opportunity to thrive.

Let's remember that supporting individuals from marginalised communities is a task that extends beyond therapy sessions. It requires advocacy, awareness, and active efforts to address systemic issues. Let us explore ways to promote inclusivity and support marginalised communities in their struggle for access to encouraging inclusivity and support marginalised communities in their effort to access quality mental health care.

Nurturing Cultural Consciousness: An Imperative Approach in Mental Health Care

It is paramount for mental health professionals to cultivate a deep understanding of cultural consciousness to provide effective and inclusive care. Take, for instance, the experience of a mental health professional supporting a transgender youth who is also part of a racial minority. The professional needs to acknowledge the intricate interplay of their clients' identities. By doing so, they can offer culturally nuanced care that addresses the specific challenges faced by transgender individuals within racial minority communities. Such an integrative approach ensures that cultural factors are considered during assessment and treatment planning, fostering an environment where the client feels genuinely acknowledged and understood.

Case Study: A mental health professional, Sarah, specialises in collaborating with immigrant communities. She takes the time to educate herself about her clients' cultural backgrounds, including their values, traditions, and languages. Through her cultural competence, Sarah creates a safe and welcoming space for her clients to discuss their mental health concerns. She tailors her therapy approaches, using culturally relevant metaphors and techniques to facilitate healing.

Amplify Marginalised Voices:

One of the most potent ways mental health professionals can advocate for marginalised communities is by amplifying their voices. By actively listening and validating their clients' experiences, mental health professionals can help individuals regain agency and self-advocacy. They can encourage clients to share their stories, promoting empowerment and raising awareness about marginalised individuals' challenges.

Case Study: Mark, a mental health counsellor, collaborates primarily with survivors of domestic violence from diverse backgrounds. Recognising the importance of amplifying their voices, Mark encourages his clients to share their experiences through art therapy, written narratives, or public speaking. He helps them develop the skills and confidence to advocate for themselves, their communities, and other abuse survivors.

Advocate for Policy Reforms:

Mental health professionals can make a significant impact by advocating for policy changes that address the systemic barriers that marginalised communities face. By collaborating with organisations focused on mental health and social justice, professionals can contribute to developing and implementing policies that promote equitable access to mental health services.

Case Study: A psychiatric nurse practitioner, Maria actively engages with local advocacy groups to address mental health disparities in underserved communities. She participates in lobbying efforts, shares her expertise in policy discussions, and writes op-eds highlighting the importance of comprehensive mental health care for marginalised populations. Through her advocacy, Maria helps implement policy changes that increase funding and improve mental health services for those in need.

Address Intersectionality:

Recognising the intersectionality of marginalised identities is crucial for mental health professionals. By understanding how various identities intersect and impact mental health, professionals can tailor treatment plans that address each client's needs and experiences.

Case Study: James, a licenced psychologist, collaborates with individuals who have experienced racial and sexual orientation-based discrimination. He acknowledges his clients' unique challenges and ensures that therapy is sensitive to their intersectional identities. James integrates trauma-informed practises, cultural rituals, and affirmative therapy approaches to help his clients navigate the complexities of their experiences.

Collaborate with Community Organisations:

Forge partnerships with community organisations serving marginalised populations to understand their specific needs better and provide targeted support. By working alongside these organisations, mental health professionals can bridge the gap between themselves and marginalised communities, fostering trust and improving access to culturally competent care.

Case Study: A social worker, Rebecca, collaborates with a local LGBTQ+ centre to provide mental health workshops and support groups. Together, they address the mental health challenges faced by LGBTQ+ individuals, including the impacts of discrimination, identity exploration, and coming out. Rebecca's collaboration ensures that her therapeutic interventions align with the needs of the community she serves.

Continuous Education and Self-Reflection:

Staying informed about current social issues, research, and best practices is essential for mental health professionals. Engaging in ongoing professional development opportunities deepens understanding of cultural competence, trauma-informed care, and anti-oppressive frameworks. Regular self-reflection on personal biases and assumptions helps improve cultural humility and sensitivity in practice.

Case Study: Michael is a licenced therapist who regularly attends conferences and seminars on cultural diversity and social justice. He actively seeks feedback from his clients and colleagues, continuously striving to improve his cultural competence. Through his dedication to ongoing education and self-reflection, Michael ensures that his therapeutic practice remains responsive to the needs of marginalised communities.

Mental health professionals are responsible for actively supporting and advocating for marginalised communities in their practice. By cultivating cultural competence, amplifying marginalised voices, advocating for policy reforms, addressing intersectionality, collaborating with community organisations, and engaging in continuous education and self-reflection, mental health professionals can significantly dismantle systemic barriers and promote equitable mental health care. Let us collectively work towards a society where mental health support is accessible, inclusive, and affirming for all individuals, regardless of their background or identity. Together, we can create meaningful change and improve the well-being of marginalised communities.

Fostering Allyship and Collaboration: Promoting Inclusivity in Mental Health Care

In our increasingly diverse and interconnected world, mental health professionals, workplaces, and society must actively foster allyship and collaboration with individuals from diverse backgrounds. Creating inclusive environments that value and celebrate diversity can significantly enhance mental health care outcomes and promote social justice. In this article, we will explore the steps that mental health professionals, workplaces, and society can take to foster allyship and collaboration, ensuring everyone receives the support they need to thrive.

Empowering Practices for Mental Health Professionals: Cultivating Cultural Competence and Promoting Inclusivity

As mental health professionals, we can substantially foster inclusivity and equality within our scope of influence. This responsibility translates into a few critical practices that we can consciously implement:

a) Fostering Cultural Consciousness: The cornerstone of empathetic and inclusive therapy is nurturing cultural consciousness. This entails a proactive approach to comprehending diverse cultures, traditions, histories, and social contexts. It necessitates introspection to identify and dispel our inherent biases, assumptions, and prejudices, which allows us to evolve continually as professionals.

Case Illustration: Dr Patel, a mental health professional, routinely participates in cultural competency workshops, solicits external supervision or consultation, and undergoes continuous self-reflection to bolster his understanding and sensitivity towards diverse cultural nuances.

b) Establishing Trust and Rapport: The cornerstone of effective therapy is the trust and rapport between a professional and their client. This relationship is built by crafting a safe, non-judgmental space wherein clients can voice their thoughts, feelings, and experiences. An empathetic ear and validation of their experiences can create a therapeutic bond crucial for progress.

Case Illustration: Sarah, a practising therapist, invests significant time in understanding her clients' cultural backgrounds, encompassing their values, beliefs, and communication styles. By recognising and affirming their experiences, she cultivates a relationship of trust and rapport.

c) Recognizing Intersectionality: An integral aspect of holistic care is the recognition of the intersectionality of individuals' identities. Intersectionality allows us to understand that a person's experiences and challenges are often influenced by the overlap of multiple social identities, such as race, gender, sexuality, and ability overlap of multiple social identities, such as race, gender, sexuality, and power, often influences a person's experiences and challenges.

Case Illustration: Dr Johnson, a therapist, is mindful of her clients' intersectional experiences. She understands that a Black transgender woman may navigate unique challenges that demand an incredibly nuanced approach to therapy.

Cultivating Allyship and Inclusion in Workplaces: Strategies and Contextual Examples

Workplaces across the UK, particularly those in the mental health sector, have a crucial role in fostering allyship and collaboration. The following are some impactful strategies complemented by relatable examples:

a) Embracing Diversity in Hiring Practices: Championing diversity and inclusion during the hiring process allows equal opportunities and invites various perspectives that can enrich the workplace environment. This is particularly crucial in mental health settings, where diverse experiences can enhance understanding and empathy.

Example: Mindful Employer, a UK-based initiative, provides employers with easier access to professionally recognised information, local support, training, and resources regarding mental health. They are committed to creating inclusive workplaces, focusing on diverse hiring practices.

b) Regular Training on Cultural Sensitivity and Unconscious Bias: Facilitating continuous training on cultural sensitivity and unconscious bias can help create a more respectful and understanding workplace environment.

Example: Virgin Atlantic, a renowned UK-based company, invests in regular cultural sensitivity and unconscious bias training as part of its commitment to diversity and inclusion. They acknowledge the value such training brings to their multicultural and international team and extend this understanding to their passenger services.

c) Encouraging Employee Support Networks: Creating employee support networks can provide a safe space for individuals from marginalised backgrounds to share their experiences and insights, contributing to an overall inclusive and supportive workplace culture.

Example: Headspace, a UK-based mental health organisation, encourages forming internal networks focused on specific identity groups such as LGBTQ+, BIPOC, and women's groups. These networks allow employees to connect, share experiences, and foster a sense of belonging within the workplace.

Societal Contributions to Inclusive Mental Health Care: Strategies and Illustrative Examples

Creating equitable mental health care systems is a collective responsibility; creating fair mental health care systems is a collective responsibility that extends beyond mental health professionals and organisations to every member of society. The following are vital actions individuals can adopt to promote inclusivity:

a) Pursuing Self-Education: Every individual can grow their understanding of mental health, cultural consciousness, and the distinct challenges experienced by marginalised communities. This quest for knowledge fosters empathy and facilitates more inclusive attitudes and behaviours.

Example: John, an ardent mental health advocate, dedicates himself to learning about the intersection of culture and mental health. He invests time in reading authoritative books, enrolling in educational webinars, and participating in courses that deepen his understanding.

b) Combatting Mental Health Stigma: Every person can contribute to diminishing mental health stigma by actively opposing discriminatory attitudes and misconceptions. Public sharing of personal journeys, endorsing mental health initiatives, and fostering open discussions can help decrease stigma and create safer spaces for others to seek help.

Example: Sarah uses her online platform to share her journey of grappling with mental health stigma and seeking therapeutic support. Her candid storytelling encourages others to do the same and underlines the necessity of normalising mental health discussions.

c) Advocating for Marginalised Communities: People can support these communities by magnifying their voices and advocating for their unique mental health needs. Listening to their experiences, validating their struggles, and actively working towards breaking down systemic barriers to mental health care are ways in which every individual can contribute.

Example: Maya, a proactive community organiser, collaborates with local mental health resources to conduct community meetings. These forums allow individuals to share their mental health experiences and propose tangible solutions to improve care access.

d) Practising Active Allyship: Individuals can leverage their privilege to stand in solidarity with marginalised voices. Active allyship involves acknowledging systemic inequities, amplifying the voices of those marginalised, and striving to dismantle barriers to mental health care.

Example: David, a white ally, persistently advocates for equal mental health care access. He writes to local policymakers, attends community meetings, and actively participates in allyship training workshops, demonstrating his commitment.

Building inclusive mental health care systems requires a collaborative effort from mental health professionals, workplaces, society, and every individual. By implementing culturally conscious practices, fostering partnerships, advocating for policy reform, and engaging in personal actions, we can establish a mental health care landscape that honours diversity and addresses the unique needs of marginalised communities. Each of us holds power to create an impact and contribute towards a more inclusive society where mental health is prioritised and supported. Together, we can transform the future of mental health care.

Building Inclusive and Equitable Mental Health Care Systems: A Collaborative Endeavour

Creating inclusive and equitable mental health care systems requires the collective effort of mental health professionals, workplaces, and society. It is crucial to recognise the barriers and disparities in accessing mental health care and take proactive steps to address them. This section will explore strategies mental health professionals, workplaces, and society can implement to foster allyship and collaboration, contributing to more inclusive and equitable mental health care systems.

Empowering Approaches for Mental Health Professionals:

Mental health professionals are vital in promoting inclusivity and equity within the mental health care system. Here are key steps they can take:

a) Culturally Consciousness Practises: Mental health professionals should continuously strive to improve their cultural consciousness, understanding the impact of cultural factors on mental health. This involves seeking training, self-reflection, and adopting culturally appropriate therapeutic approaches.

Example: Dr Nguyen regularly attends workshops and seminars on cultural consciousness, ensuring they stay updated with best practices and can provide culturally conscious care to their diverse clientele.

b) Intersectional Considerations: Mental health professionals should recognise and address the intersectional identities of individuals, acknowledging the compounding effects of multiple forms of marginalisation. This includes understanding the unique mental health challenges individuals face at the intersection of race, gender, sexuality, ability, and other identities.

Example: Therapist Sarah takes an intersectional approach in her practice, understanding how race, gender, and sexuality intersect to impact her clients' mental health and tailoring her therapeutic interventions accordingly.

c) Collaborative Partnerships: Mental health professionals should establish collaborative partnerships with professionals from diverse backgrounds and disciplines. This multidisciplinary approach can provide comprehensive care and ensure that individuals receive the necessary support.

Example: Dr Patel collaborates with social workers, community organisations, and healthcare providers to offer holistic care to underserved communities, recognising that mental health is interconnected with various social determinants.

Building Inclusivity and Allyship in Workplaces:

Workplaces are critical in cultivating inclusive and equitable mental health care systems. Here are some key measures they can adopt:

a) Embrace Diversity and Inclusion Policies: Organisations should focus on creating and executing policies that foster diversity and inclusion. This means embracing fair hiring practices that do not discriminate and cultivating a workplace culture that values the unique contributions of all employees.

Example: Barclays, a renowned UK-based global financial services company, is acknowledged for its comprehensive diversity and inclusion initiatives. The Diversity and Inclusion Committee within Barclay's champions equal representation at all levels of the organisation and supports the professional growth of underrepresented groups through focused mentorship programs.

b) Provide Mental Health Support: Organisations must prioritise employee well-being by introducing mental health support programs. These could include employee assistance programs, mental health resources, and flexible work policies to support mental health needs.

Example: Unilever, a leading multinational consumer goods company, offers a Global Employee Assistance Programme, providing confidential psychological support for employees and their families. The programme is part of a broader commitment to promoting mental health and well-being in the workplace.

c) Invest in Training and Education: Companies should commit to regular training and education programmes that raise awareness and understanding of mental health issues, cultural consciousness, and allyship. This knowledge and skillset enable employees to contribute to an inclusive and supportive work environment.

Example: Tesco, one of the UK's largest retailers, regularly conducts training sessions to promote mental health awareness and cultural sensitivity, fostering an inclusive workplace environment for all its staff members.

Community Engagement and Individual Responsibility:

Creating inclusive and equitable mental health care systems requires collective action from society. Here are essential steps society can take:

a) **Advocacy for Policy Changes:** Individuals and organisations can advocate for policies that promote mental health equity and address systemic barriers. This includes advocating for increased funding for mental health services, equitable distribution of resources, and culturally conscious care.

Example: Advocacy groups mobilise community members and collaborate with policymakers to push for policy changes that address mental health disparities, particularly in marginalised communities.

b) **Community Engagement:** Society can engage in community-based initiatives that raise awareness, reduce stigma, and increase access to mental health resources. This includes organising mental health awareness campaigns, supporting community-led mental health programmes, and fostering open dialogues.

Example: Community organisations partner with schools, local businesses, and healthcare providers to organise mental health fairs, workshops, and support groups, creating spaces for open conversations about mental health.

c) Collaborative Efforts: Society can promote collaboration among stakeholders, including mental health professionals, community leaders, and policymakers. This interdisciplinary collaboration allows for a more comprehensive approach to mental health care by addressing systemic issues and fostering lasting change.

Example: Collaboration between mental health professionals, community organisations, and policymakers leads to the development of culturally conscious mental health programmes and policies that serve the needs of diverse communities.

Building inclusive and equitable mental health care systems requires the active participation of mental health professionals, workplaces, and society. By adopting culturally responsive practises, fostering collaborative partnerships, and advocating for policy changes, we can create a mental health care landscape that values and supports individuals from all backgrounds. Together, we can contribute to a more inclusive and equitable society where everyone has equal access to the mental health care they need and deserve.

Chapter 4 Key Points:

1. **Antiracism and Allyship:** Mental health professionals and individuals are critical in

promoting antiracism, challenging oppressive systems, and creating an inclusive society.

2. **Embracing Chosen Family:** The concept of chosen family can serve as a source of support, especially for marginalised individuals. It demonstrates the power of empathy and unconditional acceptance.

3. **Power of Allyship:** Allies, particularly those in majority or dominant groups, are positioned to challenge inequality and amplify marginalised voices.

4. **Understanding Allyship:** Allyship is a continual commitment to combating oppressive systems, which requires self-reflection, education, and readiness to confront biases.

5. **Acknowledging Privilege:** Recognizing and leveraging privilege is crucial to allyship. It's not a personal failing but a systemic advantage that can be used to challenge inequality.

6. **Responsibility of Allies:** Allies must actively combat injustice, use their privileged voices to uplift marginalised individuals, and foster systemic change.

7. **The Hero's Journey of Allyship:** Joseph Campbell's concept of the Hero's Journey provides a framework for understanding the path to effective allyship, involving stages such as the call to adventure, meeting the mentor, and overcoming trials.

8. **Historical Examples of Allyship:** Historically, progress and change in oppressed communities' rights have often been facilitated by allies amplifying marginalised voices.

9. **Role of Mental Health Professionals in Advocacy:** Mental health professionals can play a pivotal role in advocating for marginalised communities and fostering culturally conscious and inclusive mental health care.

10. **Bempong Talking Therapy:** A centre committed to providing culturally conscious mental health care and inclusive therapy to Black individuals and other cultural minorities, illustrating the value of addressing intersectionality and fostering empowerment in mental health care.

11. **Cultural Consciousness in Mental Health Care:** Understanding and integrating clients' cultural backgrounds and experiences in mental health care is vital to providing effective and inclusive support.

12. **Building Inclusive and Equitable Mental Health Care Systems:** It's a collective effort involving mental health professionals, workplaces, and society, requiring strategies like culturally conscious practices, intersectional considerations, and collaborative partnerships.

"To create an inclusive workplace, we must directly combat systemic racism. Unveiling microaggressions, promoting diversity, and nurturing understanding ensures a thriving workspace for all."

- Jarell Bempong

Chapter 5

Creating Inclusive Workplaces: Addressing Racism and Prioritising Mental Health

Decoding the Influence of Systemic Racism on Workplace Mental Health

Systemic racism, deeply ingrained in social structures and institutions, significantly impacts various aspects of society, including the workplace. Examining how systemic racism manifests in the UK workplace and understanding its detrimental effects on individuals' mental well-being is crucial in addressing this issue and striving towards creating a more inclusive and equitable environment for all.

Unequal Opportunities and Career Advancement: Systemic racism in the UK workplace often results in unequal opportunities and barriers to career advancement for individuals from marginalised racial and ethnic backgrounds. Recent studies have highlighted significant disparities in employment rates, wage gaps, and access to promotions between racial minorities and their white counterparts.

According to the Race Disparity Audit conducted by the UK government in 2017, individuals from Black and minority ethnic (BAME) backgrounds are more likely to be unemployed, face pay gaps, and experience limited opportunities for career progression. These disparities contribute to frustration, reduced self-worth, and increased stress among minority employees.

Consider this Case Study: Ahmed, a highly qualified black professional, consistently outperforms his white colleagues. However, despite his qualifications and dedication, he observes his white counterparts being promoted more frequently. This disparity creates a profound sense of injustice, erodes his confidence, and negatively impacts his mental well-being.

Microaggressions and Racial Bias in Everyday Life

Microaggressions, often unnoticed yet harmful actions or comments expressing discriminatory biases, are prevalent in everyday life, especially in the workplace. These unintentional manifestations of discrimination significantly impact individuals from Black, Asian, and other minority ethnic backgrounds, including those from the LGBTQ+ community.

Common Types of Microaggressions Across Diverse Cultural Identities

Here are some frequent examples of microaggressions in diverse cultural settings:

1. **Stereotyping Ethnicity, Nationality and Sexual Orientation**

Surprising reactions towards an ethnic minority colleague's fluency in English, or offhand comments reinforcing harmful stereotypes about LGBTQ+

individuals, remind these individuals that they are perceived as 'others.' This perception negatively impacts their sense of belonging and security in the workplace.

2. Dismissive Behavior and Invalidating Identities

Minority employees may experience their contributions being overlooked in team discussions, which undervalues their input. The issue is even more pronounced for transgender or non-binary employees when their identity is dismissed by intentional misgendering.

3. Underestimating Abilities

Frequently assigning fewer challenging tasks to individuals from minority backgrounds reveals an implicit bias about their competence. Such bias limits their growth opportunities and perpetuates damaging stereotypes.

The Impact of Microaggressions on Mental Well-being

Microaggressions, rooted in deep-seated racial, cultural, and gender biases, significantly harm the mental health of marginalised employees. They create a sense of constant vigilance, causing emotional exhaustion and eroding a sense of belonging within the workplace. The Trades Union Congress (TUC) revealed in 2020 that over 70% of UK Black, Asian, and minority ethnic workers reported experiencing racial harassment or bullying at work. Such microaggressions heighten stress and psychological distress, decreasing job satisfaction and workplace engagement.

Case Study Analysis: Maria and Sam

For instance, Maria, a Latina employee, often becomes the subject of nationality or immigration jokes, undermining her confidence. Similarly, Sam, a non-binary individual, frequently experiences misgendering, leading to feelings of alienation. These day-to-day interactions negatively affect their mental well-being and job satisfaction.

Lack of Representation and Inclusive Policies

The absence of representation and inclusive policies significantly manifests systemic racism in workplaces. It contributes to feelings of invisibility, exclusion, and a lack of trust in the organisation when individuals from marginalised racial backgrounds don't see themselves reflected in leadership positions or company policies.

According to the Parker Review, in 2021, Black, Asian, and minority ethnic representation on FTSE 100 company boards was only 10.9%. This lack of representation limits the ability of racial minorities to influence policies and the organisational culture, perpetuating systemic racism.

Case Study Analysis: James

Take the case of James, a Black employee. He observes a lack of representation in senior management and a disconnect between company policies and diverse employees' experiences. As a result, he feels unheard and disregarded, leading to a diminished sense of belonging and mental distress.

Systemic Racism: The Impact on Mental Well-Being

Systemic racism in the UK workplace profoundly affects employees' mental well-being. Continuous exposure to discriminatory practices, biases, and microaggressions leads to chronic stress, anxiety, and depression. Studies have shown that workplace racial discrimination increases the risk of developing mental health disorders. The Mental Health Foundation reports that racial minority individuals in the UK are more likely to experience poor mental health outcomes due to systemic racism.

Deconstructing Systemic Racism and Cultivating Mental Well-Being in the Workplace

Constructing an inclusive and mentally healthy workplace entails a proactive approach to deconstructing systemic racism and enacting comprehensive measures. Here are essential steps organisations can take, supported by examples that embody these principles:

1. Cultivating an Inclusive Culture: Organisations should embrace diversity and inclusion, facilitating an environment where every employee feels valued, regardless of racial, ethnic, or identity background.

Example: Innocent Drinks runs regular 'Culture Clubs,' where teams focus on understanding and respecting diverse cultures and backgrounds. They also uphold robust anti-discrimination policies and empower employees to report any discrimination instances.

Benefits: This culture of inclusion enhances employee engagement, reduces attrition, and boosts overall job satisfaction.

2. Enhancing Representation:

Organisations must ensure diversity at all levels, including leadership positions. This helps employees from marginalised racial and identity backgrounds feel a sense of belonging and break down advancement barriers.

Example: Channel 4 in the UK actively promotes diversity in its leadership ranks, setting up specific diversity targets and fostering mentorship programmes that enhance the development of individuals from underrepresented groups.

Benefits: Enhanced representation results in diverse perspectives guiding decision-making processes, policies, and organisational culture, inspiring employees from all backgrounds.

3. Providing Culturally Conscious Support:

Organisations should offer employee assistance programmes and mental health support, be conscious of cultural nuances and be accessible.

Example: Mind, the mental health charity, partners with various businesses to provide culturally sensitive and confidential counselling services. They work with other organisations specialising in racial trauma to offer more comprehensive support.

Benefits: Offering such support helps employees manage systemic racism's effects, reducing stress and enhancing overall well-being.

4. Encouraging Allyship and Education: Organisations should prompt employees to become allies, educate themselves about systemic racism, and challenge challenging discriminatory practices.

Example: HSBC UK holds workshops and training sessions on systemic racism, unconscious bias, and allyship importance. They create employee resource groups encouraging dialogue and collaboration on diversity and inclusion initiatives.

Benefits: Promoting allyship and education cultivates empathy, understanding, and solidarity, enhancing collaboration and strengthening organisational culture.

5. Implementing Fair Policies and Practices: Regularly assessing HR policies, recruitment practices, and performance evaluation processes is crucial to ensure fairness and diminish bias.

Example: An exemplary case of such practices is Hallgarten & Novum Wines. I have personally witnessed their commitment to dismantling biases in recruitment during my sessions of delivering culturally conscious training across their UK estate. Under the diligent leadership of HR Manager Sara Simpson and Managing Director Andrew Bewes, the company has incorporated 'blind' recruitment practices. I distinctly remember Sara passionately explaining to the participants why deploying such a fair and inclusive strategy was imperative for their company. Hallgarten & Novum Wines also ensure regular checks on their performance evaluation criteria to uphold fairness and objectivity.

Benefits: Implementing fair policies and practices cultivates a sense of trust and fairness, attracting a diverse talent pool and nurturing a positive work environment.

By integrating these proactive measures, organisations can create a workplace that addresses systemic racism, promotes mental well-being, and fosters an inclusive environment. This benefits more than just individuals from marginalised racial backgrounds and significantly contributes to the organisation's overall growth and success.

In conclusion, systemic racism in the UK workplace has a tangible impact on the mental well-being of individuals from marginalised racial and ethnic backgrounds. Recognising the presence and effects of systemic racism is the first vital step towards creating a more inclusive, equitable, and mentally healthy workplace. Together, we can strive to create a workspace where everyone feels valued, respected, and empowered to excel.

The Impact of Racism on the Mental Health and Well-Being of Black and Cultural Minority Individuals: Navigating the Workplace and Beyond

Racism is a pervasive issue affecting societies worldwide, manifesting in various forms and settings, including the workplace. The impact of racism on the mental health and well-being of Black and cultural minority individuals is profound, leading to significant challenges and disparities. In this section, we will delve into the multifaceted effects of racism on mental health, explore its manifestations in the workplace, and discuss strategies for individuals and organisations to address these issues and foster a more inclusive and equitable environment.

Understanding Racism's Impact on Mental Health

Racism creates a hostile and stressful environment for individuals who experience it, leading to various adverse mental health outcomes. Chronic exposure to racial discrimination can increase stress, anxiety, depression, and psychological distress. The constant need to navigate racial biases, microaggressions, and stereotypes can lead to hypervigilance and emotional exhaustion, known as racial battle fatigue. Additionally, the cumulative effects of racism can contribute to racial trauma, a form of psychological injury resulting from experiences of racial discrimination, harassment, or violence.

Impact of Racism in the Workplace: The workplace is not immune to the effects of racism, as individuals from Black and cultural minority backgrounds often face unique challenges and barriers to professional growth and well-being. One of the primary manifestations of racism in the workplace is discrimination in hiring, promotions, and salary disparities, which can lead to feelings of exclusion, a lack of opportunities, and diminished self-worth. Moreover, microaggressions, or subtle racism or bias, can create a hostile work environment and negatively impact mental health.

The experience of being tokenised, where individuals from marginalised backgrounds are seen as representatives of their entire race or ethnicity, can lead to feelings of pressure, isolation, and imposter syndrome. The burden of constantly proving oneself and navigating stereotypes can be emotionally draining and detrimental to one's overall well-being. Furthermore, the lack of representation and inclusive policies within organisations can contribute to a sense of invisibility and erasure, further exacerbating the impact of racism on mental health.

Strategies for Individuals: For individuals navigating the effects of racism on their mental health in the workplace, self-care and seeking support are crucial. Developing coping mechanisms, such as mindfulness practises, therapy, and engaging in activities that promote well-being, can help individuals manage stress and build resilience. Building connections with supportive networks, both within and outside the workplace, can provide a sense of validation and understanding.

It is also essential for individuals to assert boundaries and advocate for themselves. This may involve setting clear expectations, addressing microaggressions, and seeking mentorship opportunities. By actively challenging stereotypes and engaging in self-affirmation, individuals can counteract the adverse effects of racism on their mental health and foster a positive sense of identity.

Strategies for Organisations: Organisations are pivotal in creating inclusive and equitable workplaces, prioritising all employees' mental health and well-being. Leaders and managers must commit to fostering an environment that values diversity, actively addressing racism, and promoting inclusive policies and practices. This can include initiatives such as cultural consciousness and diversity training, unconscious bias awareness programmes, and establishing reporting mechanisms for incidents of racism or discrimination.

Representation and inclusivity should be prioritised at all levels of the organisation, including leadership positions. By diversifying hiring practises, promoting mentorship programmes, and providing equal opportunities for advancement, organisations can create a sense of belonging and empowerment among employees from diverse backgrounds. Employee resource groups can also serve as platforms for dialogue, support, and advocacy, fostering a culture of inclusion and respect.

The impact of racism on the mental health and well-being of Black and cultural minority individuals in the workplace and beyond is a pressing issue that requires attention and action. By acknowledging and addressing the systemic barriers and biases that perpetuate racism, individuals and organisations can contribute to a more inclusive and equitable society. Through education, open dialogue, and proactive measures, we can create workplaces and communities where everyone feels valued, supported, and able to thrive. Together, we can challenge the detrimental effects of racism on mental health and work towards a future that embraces diversity, equality, and mental well-being for all.

Intersectional Identities in the Workplace: Overcoming Barriers and Building Hope through Authenticity, Diversity, and Inclusion

Today's world requires creating inclusive workplaces that tackle systemic racism, acknowledge neurodiversity such as dyslexia, and prioritise mental health. These elements significantly impact employees' professional development and overall well-being. This section presents firsthand experiences from self-employment and traditional employment settings, exploring the effect of systemic racism and homophobia on mental health and its interplay with dyslexia.

Charting a Path: A Personal Journey Through Intersectionality

As a self-employed psychotherapist, my journey began with confronting my complex identity, marked by being a Black gay man and living with dyslexia. Fear of rejection from potential clients due to my intersecting identities initially made me hesitant to put my picture in directories. If left unchecked, this fear could have restricted my professional growth and affected my ability to offer authentic, empathetic support to my clients.

However, I soon understood that to establish an inclusive space for my clients, I needed to face these fears and embrace my multifaceted identity required to meet these fears and embrace my multifaceted identity to establish an inclusive space for my clients. I decided to step forward authentically, embodying and presenting the intersection of my cultural background, sexual orientation, and experiences with dyslexia.

Building Bridges: The Transformative Power of Authenticity

Embracing my unique journey had a profound impact not only on my well-being but also on my well-being and the quality of support I could offer my clients. The acceptance of my identity resonated with my clients, who appreciated the empathy and understanding derived from my personal experiences. This positive response underscored the importance of authenticity and the potential to inspire and support others dealing with similar challenges.

Sharing Hope: Embracing Intersectionality in the Workplace

My journey is not unique, and I share it as a beacon of hope for others grappling with the weight of intersecting identities. Whether it's your racial background, sexual orientation, or neurodivergent conditions like dyslexia, every facet of your identity has a place and value. Recognising and honouring this intersectionality can enrich professional spaces, allowing for a broad spectrum of perspectives that resonate with diverse audiences.

A Call to Action: Fostering Inclusive Workplaces

In the context of traditional workplaces, employees like me may be grappling with the challenges of intersecting identities. Organisations must promote inclusivity and acceptance, fostering an environment where employees feel encouraged to be authentic. This kind of setting does not just benefit employees on a personal level but contributes to a healthier, more productive, and innovative professional environment.

In conclusion, addressing systemic racism, embracing neurodiversity, and prioritising mental health are imperative in today's workplaces. We can create genuinely inclusive workplaces by fostering environments that celebrate authenticity, actively dismantle systemic barriers, and promote mental well-being. We want to create genuinely inclusive workplaces by fostering environments that celebrate authenticity, actively dismantle systemic barriers, and promote mental well-being. My story is a testament to the power of this approach, and I hope it inspires individuals and organisations alike to strive for such inclusivity.

Representation and Breaking Barriers: A Personal Triumph Over Systemic Racism Homophobia and Dyslexia

Systemic racism often manifests through a lack of representation and unequal opportunities for individuals from marginalised racial and ethnic backgrounds.

In my ongoing entrepreneurial journey, I continually encounter and strive to overcome the formidable challenge of underrepresentation. I steadfastly refuse to let these barriers define or constrain me. Instead, I actively seek a diverse clientele, persistently invest in lifelong learning to enhance my understanding, and tirelessly challenge prevailing biases. My mission is to amplify the often silenced voices from marginalised communities and to marginalised communities' often silenced voices and construct an inclusive practice where every client, regardless of their background, feels acknowledged, understood, and appreciated.

In the broader spectrum of traditional employment, it's imperative that organisations consciously work towards dismantling systemic racism by ardently promoting diversity and inclusion. This involves adopting diverse hiring practices, providing mentorship programs, creating and adopting various hiring practices, providing mentorship programs, and creating advancement opportunities for individuals from marginalised backgrounds, all within an inclusive workplace culture. In an environment where everyone feels valued and represented, the collective diversity of perspectives and experiences can be leveraged, driving innovation, creativity, and organisational growth.

Strength through Adversity: Overcoming Discrimination and Harnessing Inner Dragons for Growth and Inclusion

Mental health issues, traumas, and challenges are mighty dragons in our psychological landscapes. As a self-employed psychotherapist, I navigate this terrain, engaging with these symbolic creatures. I've learned that these dragons, emblematic of our adversities, can become allies. Their formidable power and fiery might become a force for illumination, shedding light on obscured aspects of our psyche and illuminating the boundless potential for personal growth within each of us.

One such adversity many of us face is systemic racism and discrimination. Its impact is like a pervasive dragon whose fiery breath scorches the fields of our professional lives and whose presence casts a long shadow on our mental well-being. Yet, in the face of this formidable adversary, I have seen resilience and triumph that have become sources of strength and inspiration for me and others.

By sharing these stories, I aim to embolden others to embrace their identities, challenge bias, and pursue their passions without fear. Recognising systemic racism as the dragon it is, we can rally our collective strength to address and challenge its presence in self-employment and traditional employment settings. This collective confrontation can create empowering work environments championing diversity, inclusivity, and mental well-being.

In the workplace, those who have experienced discrimination can harness their adversities, turning their experiences into a source of strength and motivation to advocate for change. They become dragon-tamers and not slayers, using their experiences to share stories, raise awareness, and collaborate with colleagues and leadership. Their endeavours create an inclusive workplace culture where diversity is celebrated, and all voices are valued.

I believe in fostering an environment of inclusion and prioritising mental well-being, and as a psychotherapist, I make this a cornerstone of my practice. Through equitable policies, challenging biases, and promoting diversity, I aim to create a supportive environment where all feel they belong. Such an inclusive environment enhances individuals' mental well-being, encouraging professional growth and benefiting the broader work environment.

In traditional employment settings, organisations can prioritise mental health by implementing employee assistance programs, providing diversity and inclusion training, and establishing open, honest communication channels. These supportive structures and a culture of empathy can counteract the negative impact of systemic racism on mental well-being.

In conclusion, systemic racism, in both self-employment and traditional employment settings, has far-reaching effects on individuals' mental well-being and professional experiences. Through my practice as a psychotherapist and interactions with diverse workplaces, I've observed the transformative power of facing fear, embracing authenticity, and fostering inclusion.

The dragons of systemic racism are formidable but not invincible. By acknowledging and challenging these dragons, individuals and organisations can create workplaces that celebrate diversity, prioritise mental health, and provide equal opportunities for everyone to thrive. Together, we can forge a more inclusive and equitable future. We will not merely slay the dragons but tame them, transforming their fiery presence into a force for change and growth. By doing so, no individual will be limited or excluded based on race, ethnicity, or other aspects of their identity. Everyone can bring their whole selves to work, having harnessed the might of their inner dragons to illuminate the path ahead.

Culturally Conscious Approaches to Mental Well-Being: Integrative Strategies for Organisations

In mental health, organisations are significant in nurturing an environment of culturally conscious well-being. By integrating various therapeutic modalities such as Person-centred Centred Therapy, Culturally Conscious Therapy, Trauma-based Therapy, Rational Emotive Behavioural Therapy (REBT), Neuro Neuro-Linguistic Programming (NLP), Cognitive Behavioural Therapy (CBT), Narrative Therapy, Mindfulness-Based Therapy, they can proactively support and guide individuals on their healing journey.

1. **Creating a culture of cultural consciousness among staff members is a critical first step for organisations.** This means fostering an environment that values diversity and inclusivity and implementing training programmes encouraging dialogue and cross-cultural understanding. For example, comprehensive cultural competency training can equip mental health professionals with the necessary skills to provide culturally sensitive care, ensuring clients from diverse backgrounds feel heard, understood, and respected.

2. **The adaptation of culturally sensitive assessment tools is also essential. These** tools gather comprehensive information about clients' mental health and specific needs while considering their cultural backgrounds. Such tools can help organisations tailor treatment plans to address clients' unique experiences and cultural nuances.

3. **Therapeutic approaches must also include cultural sensitivity**. This means integrating clients' cultural values, beliefs, and practices into therapeutic modalities. By doing so, organisations can create a therapeutic space that is inclusive, respectful, and tailored to each individual's unique cultural context.

4. **Culturally adapted interventions that address individuals' specific needs and challenges from diverse backgrounds are equally crucial.** By incorporating cultural values, beliefs, and practices into therapy sessions, organisations can ensure that the therapeutic journey is practical and respectful of each individual's cultural identity.

5. **Education and raising awareness also play a vital role. Providing** educational resources

covering various mental health topics and cultural issues can increase awareness, reduce stigma, and empower individuals to engage actively in their mental well-being. These resources can foster a holistic understanding of well-being that recognises the intersectionality of mental health and culture.

6. **Organisations should also create safe, inclusive spaces for individuals from diverse backgrounds to share their experiences and learn from one another.** This could include support groups and workshops encouraging dialogue, healing, and personal growth. These gatherings offer culturally sensitive support and promote resilience within a safe and inclusive environment.

7. **Supplementing therapy with culturally sensitive self-help materials, such as workbooks, worksheets, guided meditations, or relaxation exercises, can reinforce the skills learned during therapy sessions.** These resources empower individuals to engage in self-care and personal growth beyond the therapy room.

8. **Lastly, organisations should establish referral networks comprising trusted professionals and organisations specialising in areas outside their expertise.** This collaborative approach ensures that clients receive comprehensive care that meets their diverse needs.

These strategies can help organisations promote a culturally conscious approach to mental well-being. By supporting individuals from diverse cultural backgrounds and fostering inclusive and empowering environments, organisations can contribute significantly to promoting healing, growth, and resilience. Together, we can work towards making mental well-being accessible and relevant to everyone, regardless of their cultural identity.

Beyond Symbolic Gestures: Advancing Culturally Conscious Mental Well-being

In the quest for culturally conscious mental well-being, the difference between organisations that deeply invest in this imperative and those that resort to symbolic or performative acts is stark. It is one thing to post a black square on Instagram in solidarity with Black Lives Matter (BLM) and another to dismantle systemic biases and foster inclusivity within an organisation actively. This distinction illuminates the chasm between superficial gestures and genuine commitment to advancing mental health care for individuals from diverse cultural backgrounds.

This contrast is particularly evident when examining the disparities in approaches taken by organisations and practitioners. On the one hand, some organisations recognise the necessity of moving beyond lip service, understanding that meaningful engagement with cultural consciousness is integral to their mission. They diligently work to raise awareness, educate their workforce, and implement culturally conscious practices. In the case of mental health care, organisations often employ a multi-modal therapeutic approach, incorporating techniques such as Person-centred Therapy, Culturally Conscious Therapy, Trauma-based Therapy, Rational Emotive Behavioural Therapy, Neuro Neuro-Linguistic Programming,

Cognitive Behavioural Therapy, Narrative Therapy, Mindfulness-Based Therapy.

Within these organisations, therapy isn't one-size-fits-all; it's adapted to acknowledge and respect each cultural context's unique experiences. Such is the approach at Bempong Talking Therapy Ltd., where the focus is not merely on culturally conscious care but also on creating a diverse, inclusive environment and a therapeutic space tailored to each individual's needs and background.

On the other hand, some organisations may engage in performative allyship, using symbolic gestures such as posting a black square on Instagram for BLM, yet failing to follow through with substantive actions. In contrast, such acts may communicate support without concurrent and sustained efforts to address systemic racism and promote cultural inclusivity within the organisation; these gestures risk being perceived as hollow.

Fostering culturally conscious mental well-being demands more than performative allyship or surface-level diversity and inclusion initiatives. It requires a deep, authentic commitment to understand and respect the cultural nuances that shape individuals' mental health experiences.

By recognising the significance of this commitment, organisations can move beyond symbolic gestures, cultivate a genuinely inclusive environment, and provide practical, culturally conscious mental health support. The journey towards culturally conscious mental well-being is ongoing, requiring persistent efforts and genuine engagement from all stakeholders in the mental health field.

Impact of Authentic Commitment and Superficial Gestures on Culturally Conscious Mental Well-being

1. The Role of Authentic Organisations:

Organisations like Mind, a UK-based mental health charity, are committed to cultural sensitivity and inclusivity. By incorporating diversity into their work, they offer a supportive environment for individuals from different cultural backgrounds. This approach contributes to better mental health outcomes and a more inclusive society.

2. Superficial Efforts and Their Consequences:

Some organisations focus more on appearances, treating cultural consciousness as a superficial gesture. This lack of depth leaves systemic issues unresolved, failing to provide support for individuals from diverse backgrounds and slowing societal progress towards equity.

3. Limited Training Initiatives:

Short-term training initiatives are a common feature of organisations focusing on appearance over substance. These efforts, lacking depth and continuity, need to cultivate a culture of empathy and acceptance. This deficiency leaves individuals feeling unsupported and perpetuates societal difficulties in handling cultural diversity.

4. Inadequate Resources:

Superficially focused organisations often fail to provide adequate resources for culturally sensitive mental health care. This shortfall affects the well-being of individuals relying on these services and widens societal disparities. Genuine commitment, as shown by the UK's Equality and Human Rights Commission, requires consistent effort and learning.

5. Authentic Commitment:

We promote a societal shift towards diversity and mental well-being by supporting authentic organisations like Mind or the Equality and Human Rights Commission. This commitment brings positive change, fostering a society that respects cultural differences and promotes mental health.

6. Collaborating for Impact:

Authentic organisations often work with socially responsible partners to create inclusive environments. These collaborations enhance the mental well-being of individuals from all cultural backgrounds and move society towards greater inclusivity.

7. Leading by Example:

Organisations like the Mental Health Foundation and the Time to Change campaign demonstrate steadfast commitment to culturally conscious mental well-being. These organisations provide resources, education, and interventions that respect and respond to cultural differences. By supporting these organisations, we can contribute to a more inclusive society that values cultural diversity and promotes mental health for all.

In conclusion, the difference between organisations that genuinely commit to fostering culturally conscious mental well-being and those that engage in superficial gestures is profound. This distinction holds significant implications for individuals' mental health, society's understanding and acceptance of cultural diversity, and our collective progress towards equity and inclusivity. By actively supporting organisations that demonstrate a genuine commitment to cultural consciousness, we contribute to a more inclusive, equitable society that values and nurtures mental well-being for all, regardless of cultural identity. Hence, the emphasis should be on consistent actions that challenge systemic biases, promote understanding, and offer comprehensive, culturally conscious mental health support. Only then can we collectively achieve a society where cultural diversity is appreciated, respected, and integrated into the mental health sphere.?

Championing Change: A Comprehensive Guide to Battling Workplace Discrimination and Fostering Mental Health in the UK"

Navigating the intricacies of workplace discrimination and advocating for mental health can be intimidating. But fear not. This comprehensive guide aims to empower those affected by these issues and those willing to stand as their allies with the knowledge and tools necessary to confront these challenges head-on. This is more than a mere journey; it is a proactive stand against discrimination and a crucial step towards cultivating an inclusive and equitable work environment. You'll find valuable strategies through the comprehensive insights shared in this guide. These will equip you to foster healthier, compassionate, and understanding workplaces, thus transforming them into safe havens of acceptance and respect. This odyssey, while formidable, is one we can undertake together, turning daunting into achievable.

1. **Learn and Understand: Understanding begins with knowledge:** Learn about different forms of discrimination and how mental health issues may present themselves. The Equality Act 2010 in the UK offers legal protections for individuals with mental health conditions considered disabilities. Being informed of your rights empowers you to identify and challenge injustices, creating a safer, more equitable workspace.

2. **Look After Yourself: Ensuring your mental health is a cornerstone of this journey:** Exercise regularly, maintain a balanced diet, sleep well, and practice mindfulness. All these habits build resilience and contribute to your overall mental health. The NHS offers Cognitive Behavioural Therapy (CBT) in the UK, an invaluable resource for professional help and coping strategies.

3. **Talk Openly:** Open communication fosters an understanding and supportive work environment. Expressing your mental health needs to your employer helps create a tailored approach to your well-being. The Disability Confident Scheme and Employee Assistance Programmes (EAPs) in the UK

offer supportive resources, including counselling services.

4. **Ask for Adjustments:** If your mental health condition is considered a disability under the Equality Act, you're entitled to reasonable adjustments at work. These can be flexible hours, working from home, or regular breaks. Advocating for these adjustments ensures a work environment conducive to your mental well-being.

5. **Document Incidents:** Recording instances of discrimination provides crucial evidence if you decide to complain. This written account can prove indispensable in effecting workplace change and holding perpetrators accountable.

6. **Speak Up:** Report instances of discrimination to your organisation's relevant authority. If the issue persists, contact the UK's external bodies, such as the Advisory, Conciliation and Arbitration Service (ACAS) or the Equality and Human Rights Commission (EHRC). Speaking up transforms you from a passive observer to an active catalyst for change.

7. **Find Support:** Joining support groups, whether within your workplace or externally, within your workplace or externally, provides a safe space for shared experiences. This supportive network can offer practical advice, emotional support, and a sense of community.

8. **Get Professional Help:** If your mental health is severely affected, seek professional assistance. The NHS offers mental health services in

the UK, including talk therapies and dedicated mental health teams.

9. **Push for Change:** Advocating for mental health training, anti-discrimination policies, and secure reporting channels in your workplace creates systemic change. Your voice can significantly contribute to fostering an environment that respects mental health and treats everyone fairly.

Even if you're not personally affected by workplace discrimination or mental health struggles, you can make your workplace a safer, more supportive environment. As an ally, your journey will involve listening, learning, and supporting those who need it.

Unleashing the Power of Solidarity: A Transformative Guide to Becoming an Unwavering Ally

1. **Education and Awareness:** As an ally, your first responsibility is to educate yourself. Understand the myriad forms of discrimination and mental health conditions. Knowing the protections provided by laws like the Equality Act 2010 in the UK can be immensely helpful when advocating for those affected.

2. **Promote Self-Care:** Encourage colleagues to engage in self-care practices that foster mental well-being. Your support can create an environment where mental health is prioritised and not stigmatised. Remind your co-workers about resources such as the Cognitive Behavioural Therapy (CBT) offered by the NHS in the UK.

3. **Encourage Open Communication:** Foster an atmosphere where your colleagues can openly discuss their mental health needs. Advocate for using resources such as the Disability Confident Scheme and Employee Assistance Programmes (EAPs) in the UK.

4. **Support Reasonable Adjustments:** If a colleague has a mental health condition classified as a disability under the Equality Act, they are eligible for workplace adjustments. Please support them in requesting adjustments, such as flexible working hours, remote work, or regular breaks.

5. **Help Document Incidents**: If a colleague experiences discrimination, assist them in documenting the incident. Your support can provide the courage and resources they need to act further.

6. **Stand Up Against Discrimination:** If you witness discrimination, report it. Your voice can lend much-needed support to a colleague and push the organisation to take action. If necessary, support your colleague in contacting external bodies like the UK's Advisory, Conciliation and Arbitration Service (ACAS) or the Equality and Human Rights Commission (EHRC).

7. **Foster a Supportive Network:** Actively participate in or help establish support groups within your workplace. These groups can offer a haven for colleagues to share experiences and find allies. These platforms also allow you to learn more about their struggles and how you can support them effectively.

8. **Encourage Seeking Professional Help:** If a colleague's mental health is severely

affected, encourage them to seek professional help. Remind them that services are available, like those offered by the NHS in the UK, including talking therapies and mental health teams.

9. **Advocate for Systemic Change:** Push your workplace to implement mental health training, comprehensive anti-discrimination policies, and secure avenues for reporting instances of discrimination. Your advocacy can instigate a systemic change that fosters a more inclusive and understanding work environment.

As we navigate the complex cultural crossroads, dismantling racism and promoting equity in mental health care and beyond requires a deep understanding of the interconnectedness of our identities and experiences. As I confronted my misconceptions about Africa and found empowerment through self-acceptance and resilience, individuals can contribute to this vital work by actively embracing cultural consciousness.

To dismantle systemic racism and promote equity, it is crucial to celebrate and respect diverse experiences; I often say, "In embracing cultural consciousness, we foster a world where diverse experiences are celebrated and respected."

Recognising and challenging the skewed narratives and harmful stereotypes that permeate society is essential. This includes confronting the legacies of colonialism, white supremacy, and social biases that have shaped our collective understanding of history and identity. By actively seeking out and amplifying marginalised voices, we can reshape the narrative to be more inclusive and accurate.

Education plays a pivotal role in this process. By critically examining the curriculum and materials taught in schools, universities, and other educational institutions, we can ensure that they represent diverse perspectives and histories, free from biased portrayals. Moreover, educating ourselves and others about the complexities of different cultures and accounts can lead to a more informed and compassionate society.

In promoting equity in mental health care, we must recognise the intersectionality of identities and experiences. Mental health care should be culturally conscious and responsive to the unique needs of individuals from diverse backgrounds. This includes challenging stigmas and stereotypes associated with mental health in various cultures and ensuring that mental health services are accessible and inclusive.

Beyond mental health care, promoting equity requires fostering inclusive workplaces and communities. Individuals can advocate for diversity and inclusion in their workplaces, challenge discriminatory practices, and support policies that address systemic inequalities. By actively engaging in conversations about race, identity, and social justice, individuals can create safe spaces for open dialogue and learning.

Allyship is also a crucial aspect of dismantling racism and promoting equity. Supporting and amplifying the voices of marginalised individuals, actively standing against racism and discrimination, and using one's privilege to uplift others are all powerful ways to contribute to positive change.

Ultimately, this journey towards dismantling racism and promoting equity in mental health care and beyond requires collective action. Each individual's efforts, no matter how small, can contribute to the larger goal of creating a more just and inclusive world. By acknowledging the complexities of our identities and working together with empathy and compassion, we can make meaningful strides towards a brighter, more equitable future for all.

Chapter 5 Key Points:

1. Systemic Racism and Its Implications: Systemic racism in the UK workplace leads to unequal opportunities, wage gaps, and career advancement barriers, affecting individuals from minority racial and ethnic backgrounds. The Race Disparity Audit revealed significant disparities and their adverse impact on minority employees' mental well-being.

2. Microaggressions and Mental Health: Microaggressions stemming from racial, cultural, and gender biases harm the mental health of marginalised employees. Many Black, Asian, and minority ethnic workers reported racial harassment or bullying, increasing stress and psychological distress.

3. Systemic Racism and Mental Well-being: The UK workplace's systemic racism profoundly affects employees' mental health. Chronic exposure to discriminatory practices and biases leads to stress, anxiety, and depression, increasing the risk of developing mental health disorders.

4. Cultivating Mental Well-being in the Workplace: Constructing an inclusive and mentally healthy workplace requires dismantling systemic racism, acknowledging neurodiversity, and prioritising mental health. Personal narratives and case studies show the benefits of authenticity, diversity, and inclusion in overcoming systemic barriers.

5. Culturally Conscious Approaches to Mental Well-being: Organisations play a pivotal role in fostering culturally conscious mental well-being. Organisations can support individuals on their healing journey by incorporating various therapeutic modalities and promoting cultural consciousness.

6. Authentic Commitment vs Superficial Gestures: Genuine commitment to cultural consciousness and inclusivity leads to better mental health outcomes, whereas superficial gestures and limited initiatives leave systemic issues unresolved and fail to provide adequate support.

7. A Comprehensive Guide to Battling Workplace Discrimination: The guide empowers individuals with knowledge and tools to confront discrimination and advocate for mental health. It includes understanding legal protections, maintaining mental health, open communication, supporting workplace adjustments, and reporting discrimination.

In embracing cultural consciousness, we foster a world where diverse experiences are celebrated and respected.

Jarell Bempong.

Chapter 6

Dismantling Racism, Promoting Mental Health: Empowering Individuals for Change

Resilience Amid Bias: Confronting Colonialism and White Supremacy in Ghana and Britain

Within the confines of an all-English elementary school, my identity was shaped and confined by the limited perspectives around me. As one of the few Black students, I was swayed by the narrative, finding solace in the Jamaican heritage claimed by the only other Black boys in my school. Unknowingly, I was immersed in a cultural echo chamber where Africa was projected as a monolithic entity, a primitive land with no history beyond slavery, and a wild place inhabited solely by exotic animals and enslaved peoples.

Stitched into this web of skewed perceptions were tales of Africans being responsible for the slave trade. Such stories were cruelly whispered into the ears of impressionable minds, mine included. They were underpinned by an accusation as sharp as a sword's edge, blaming Africans for the trials and tribulations of Caribbean people. The harmful stereotype of the African as primitive and backwards was cemented within me, causing me to subconsciously distance myself from this African identity, even leading me to embrace a Jamaican identity that I mistook as my own.

These misconceptions that misconceptions I held about Africa were not solely perpetuated by schoolyard chatter. They were reaffirmed by the narrative of Empire and history taught in school, depicted in movies, and subtly woven into the fabric of our society.

Then, one ordinary day, my perception of self was upended by my mother's simple yet earth-shattering revelation: "You are Ghanaian!"

This newfound knowledge marked a pivotal shift in my understanding of self. The journey of self-discovery propelled me and led me to confront my true heritage when I had to relocate to Ghana with my family. Suddenly, I stood at the crossroads of my rich cultural heritage and the stark realities of colonialism, white supremacy, and deeply entrenched societal biases.

In this personal account, I dive into the convoluted intersections of identity, race, mental health, queerness, and dyslexia. I explore the myriad ways these facets of my being were coloured by the insidious spectres of white supremacy and colourism and how the oppressive nature of societal norms seeped into my experiences.

Join me as I navigate the treacherous waters of my personal history, peel back layers of adversity, and find empowerment through self-acceptance and resilience. This is my tale of transformation as a British-Ghanaian, a story of negotiating the complex cultural crossroads of Ghana and England, reconciling deep-seated misconceptions with my true heritage, and finding strength within the heart of adversity. This is a story of resilience amid colonialism, neocolonialism, white supremacy, and societal biases. This story lays bare the multi-layered nature of our identities, unfolding a narrative that goes far beyond the monolithic portrayals of Africa.

Arriving in Ghana: The Reflective Mirror of Society and Colourism:

As we descended into our new life in Ghana, I began to see our diverse family as a microcosm of society - a complex tapestry woven with various threads of identity. With a Ghanaian mother, a white English stepfather, an older Black brother, and two biracial siblings, our family portrait reflected the intersections of race, colour, and culture. It mirrored the societal dynamics in this land, where the remnants of colonialism and the pervasive influence of white supremacy were all too evident.

It wasn't long before I came face-to-face with the deeply entrenched colourism that lurked within the folds of Ghanaian society. This was a world where lighter skin was celebrated, where people bleached it to escape the societal disdain that came with a darker complexion. I noticed the preferential treatment my younger siblings received due to their lighter skin, both within our home and in the broader society.

Among the most potent manifestations of white supremacy was the white saviour mentality that people attached to my stepfather. They flocked around him as if he were their redeemer, their Messiah who would pull them from their predicaments. The implicit message was devastating: he, with his white skin, was superior to us, his own family.

I found myself grappling with an array of emotions as I processed these experiences. Feelings of alienation, frustration, and resentment swirled within me. The sting of being sidelined, the bitter pill of feeling less than - these were experiences that clung to me, shaping my understanding of the world and my place within it. I was standing at the crossroads of my Blackness and the omnipresent spectre of white supremacy. It was a harsh awakening to the realities of colourism and an uneasy negotiation with my queerness in a society where such identities were often met with hostility.

As I navigated through these tumultuous waters, my understanding of myself and the world around me evolved knowledge of myself and the world around me grew as I navigated through these turbulent waters. It was an arduous journey of resilience, self-discovery, and growth. Through my experiences, I began to see the insidious effects of white supremacy and colourism. I understood the societal pressures that drove people to bleach their skin and the pervasive sense of inferiority that haunted those of us with darker skin.

This narrative seeks to shed light on these complexities, unveiling the pervasive nature of white supremacy and colourism within society and how they intersect with our identities. It explores the emotional terrain of feeling sidelined, the struggle for self-acceptance, and the power of resilience in the face of adversity. It's a journey through the cultural landscape of Ghana and Britain and a reflection on the layered nature of identity amid colonialism, white supremacy, and societal biases.

Unearthing Hidden Narratives: Navigating Abrahamic Religion, Patriarchy, Homophobia, and Ghana's Queer Legacies

I was tangled in layers of oppression, from white supremacy and colonialism to colourism and homophobia. On top of these, the strict rules of a deeply rooted patriarchy also ensnared me. As if these challenges weren't enough, whitewashed religious teachings fuelled intense homophobia in Ghanaian society.

Distorted religious beliefs, shaped by a colonial past, led to a deep fear of punishment from God and rejection by society. This silenced any talk about LGBTQ+ identities. Trapped in this complex discrimination network, my journey to fully accept and celebrate my authentic self felt daunting and almost impossible.

However, amidst this turbulent period, I stumbled upon a part of our history that challenged these beliefs. As I dug deeper into my Ghanaian heritage, I re-discovered the 'ObaaBarima'. This term, 'woman-man', is used in traditional Ghanaian society to recognise a third-gender identity. It is a testament to gender fluidity, long before the Western world acknowledged or validated it.

In pre-colonial times, 'ObaaBarima' was respected in their communities. They served as seers, mediators, and healers. Their ability to challenge rigid gender norms gave them a special place in society. This challenges the belief that queerness was 'un-African' or a 'Western' concept.

In today's Ghana, 'ObaaBarima' is still present. They're often misunderstood as men brought up by women. They're seen as funny, nurturing, and sociable, often spending time with women. Their charming and friendly nature wins them the affection of the community. But these perceptions also undermine the profound significance of the 'ObaaBarima' identity, reducing it to comedy and charm.

I'm not saying my sexuality is the same as the gender fluidity that 'ObaaBarima' represents. However, the fact that such an identity is recognised and accepted in society shows that diversity and fluidity in gender and sexual identities were a part of pre-colonial African societies.

This deep dive into the hidden aspects of queerness in Ghanaian heritage sparked a sense of validation and empowerment within me. It provided a new perspective, different from the repressive ideologies I'd been wrestling with. It served as a reminder that our struggles are not inherent. They result from systems and constructs that can - and should - be challenged and reformed.

An Unexpected Beacon: Mrs Joan Ofori, My Ally in a Dyslexic World

Navigating dyslexia in an unsupportive environment was a daunting challenge. Adding to this struggle was the constant comparison to my academically gifted older brother, leaving me feeling inadequate and labelled as unintelligent.

Amidst these difficulties, Mrs Joan Ofori emerged as an unexpected source of hope. A White

English headmistress who had moved to Ghana for love, she became a pivotal figure in my life, identifying and helping me with dyslexia.

Under her guidance, I explored innovative learning techniques, like tracing words on paper and using tactile interactions to grasp spellings. Her methods were transformative and provided a lifeline in a world that often misunderstood dyslexia.

Sadly, Mrs Ofori's passing left me without support once again. Yet, her impact on my life went beyond the classroom. She empowered me to recognise my potential and gave me the tools to overcome societal barriers.

Today, I am a testament to resilience; despite dropping out of university two despite dropping out of university twice, I am a testament to strength. Discovering diplomas as my preferred mode of education, I made up for lost time, collecting credentials that bolstered my knowledge and skills. In this book, I share the knowledge gained from my experiences, aiming to empower others to overcome challenges and discover their true potential.

Finding My Place: From Struggles to Self-Expression in the UK

My return to England was a change of scene that marked a critical transition in my life. At this stage, where multiculturalism and acceptance of diversity flourished, I found the support and resources needed to truly understand and embrace myself: my Ghanaian heritage, my blackness, my queerness, and my neurodivergence.

However, the journey was challenging. Adjusting to life in the UK took time and involved dealing with unexpected obstacles. I share Some of these trials with you in this book, while others might be tales for another text or an intriguing conversation over coffee.

Once I navigated these initial hurdles, I found a liberating environment devoid of the constraints of homophobia, colourism, and ableism I had previously encountered. This liberation allowed me to blossom and tap into my untapped creative potential. Amid this newfound freedom, I discovered my passion for writing, a vehicle for sharing my unique perspective.

Tying the Threads: Navigating Challenges and Thriving Amid Diversity:

Over time, my journey across continents, from Ghana to the UK, has been riddled with both challenges and triumphs. Amid navigating the complexities of colonialism, white supremacy, colourism, homophobia, and dyslexia, I have steadily found my footing and, more importantly, begun to thrive. Each obstacle I have surmounted has added to my resilience, and those hard-learned lessons have given birth to this book.

An Advocate for Intersectionality: Amplifying Voices from the Margins:

My multifaceted journey has highlighted the pressing need for intersectional advocacy. My experiences aren't unique but mirror those of countless others at the intersection of multiple identities. By penning my journey, I aim to amplify the voices of those often marginalised, challenge ingrained societal norms, and dismantle oppressive systems. My fervent hope is to foster inclusivity and equity and, in the process, nudge the world towards understanding, empathy, and education. These essential steps can lay the foundation for a compassionate world where individuals can celebrate their authentic selves.

A Look Back and a Step Forward:

Reflecting on my journey, spanning the breadth of my experiences from embracing Ghanaian culture to navigating the impacts of white supremacy, colourism, homophobia, and the challenges posed by dyslexia, I am reminded of the extraordinary resilience within each of us. Despite the multitude of adversities, I have emerged more robust more empowered, and with a fierce passion for utilising adversities, I have emerged more muscular, more empowered, and with an intense passion for using my voice to effect positive change.

By acknowledging and actively dismantling the intersecting systems of oppression, we can shape a world that truly values and uplifts every individual, irrespective of race, sexuality, skin colour, or neurodivergence. As we move forward, let's work together to pave the way for a future where every person can embrace their true self. This dream for an inclusive, equitable society isn't just possible - it's within our grasp. Let us each play our part in making it a reality.

Individual Contributions to Dismantling Systemic Racism and Promoting Equity:

To dismantle systemic racism and promote equity in mental health care and beyond, individuals play a crucial role. Recognising the pervasive nature of white supremacy, and other discriminatory power dynamics, individuals can actively contribute in several ways:

Education and Awareness:

- Engage in self-education about white supremacy's historical context and manifestations.
- Learn about significant dates and events, such as the civil rights movement in the United States, anti-apartheid movements, and other struggles for racial justice globally.
- Raise awareness among peers, family, and community about systemic racism and discrimination and its impact on mental health.

Allyship and Advocacy:

- Stand in solidarity with marginalised communities, amplify their voices, and actively challenge discriminatory practices.
- Advocate for policies that promote equity and inclusion in mental health care, education, and employment.

- Support organisations that work towards dismantling systemic racism and discrimination and addressing mental health disparities.

Cultivate Cultural Consciousness:

- Seek to understand diverse cultures, perspectives, and experiences.

Challenge and unlearn biases and stereotypes:

- Embrace cultural diversity in mental health care practices and ensure culturally conscious approaches that address the unique needs of marginalised communities.

Promote Representation and Inclusion:

- Advocate for increased representation of people of colour in positions of power and decision-making, including within mental health institutions, research, and policymaking.
- Push for inclusive hiring practices that combat discrimination and promote diversity.

Support Grassroots Movements:

- Contribute time, resources, or donations to grassroots organisations that actively work towards dismantling systemic racism, advancing social justice, and addressing mental health disparities within marginalised communities.

Self-reflection and Personal Growth:

- Engage in introspection and acknowledge personal biases and privileges.
- Continuously work on becoming an anti-racist individual by challenging and unlearning harmful beliefs and behaviours.

Dismantling systemic racism and promoting equity in mental health care requires collective effort and individual commitment. By understanding the historical origins, global impact, and devastating consequences of white supremacy, individuals can take tangible steps to combat systemic racism. Individuals contribute to creating a more equitable and inclusive society through education, allyship, advocacy, cultural competence, and supporting grassroots movements. By addressing mental health disparities and dismantling the structures perpetuating inequality, individuals can foster a sense of belonging, empowerment, and well-being for marginalised communities.

The Kitchen Chronicles: Embracing Cultural Consciousness in Therapy

As a budding therapist, my journey was not without its challenges. Being a Black, dyslexic man in a field dominated by white, neurotypical professionals, I often felt like an outlier. Amidst the diversity of psychology diploma courses, I was frequently the only

Gay student, further adding to my sense of being out of place. However, I was determined to make a difference in people's lives, and it was during a practice therapy session that a transformative moment occurred.

A Pivotal Moment of Reflection:

Playing the role of the therapist, I engaged in a practice therapy session with my fellow student, Emily. As she shared her kitchen renovation experience, I became enthralled and fascinated by her storytelling. In my excitement, I made an assumption about her relationship and mistakenly referred to excitedly, I assumed her relationship and mistakenly referred to her partner as her husband. However, I quickly realised she was a lesbian, and the person in question was her wife. In that instant, embarrassment washed over me, mainly as I was gay.

An Immediate and Authentic Apology:

Recognising my mistake, I swiftly offered an authentic apology, expressing my sincere regret for making assumptions rooted in societal norms and gender stereotypes. I explained that my intention was never to misrepresent or invalidate her relationship. My heartfelt apology came from understanding the importance of cultural consciousness and the impact of my words on her.

Learning from Mistakes:

This pivotal moment of reflection taught me a profound lesson. We all hold biases and misconceptions, often unknowingly perpetuating harmful assumptions. However, it is our responsibility to learn from our mistakes, apologise sincerely, and work we are responsible for learning from our mistakes, apologising sincerely, and working towards challenging and dismantling our biases. As a therapist, I realised that being culturally conscious was an ongoing journey of self-awareness and empathy.

A Commitment to Growth:

In the aftermath of the incident, I dedicated myself to educating myself about diverse experiences and perspectives. I engaged in conversations, sought resources, and deepened my understanding of LGBTQ+ issues. This commitment to growth enabled me to create a safe and inclusive space for my clients where they felt respected and seen.

The Kitchen Chronicles was a transformative experience in my journey as a therapist. The embarrassment of my mistaken assumption led to an immediate and authentic apology, where I acknowledged my biases and misconceptions. I learned the importance of cultural consciousness, recognising that we all have blind spots that require introspection and empathy. Today, I strive to create a world where diversity is celebrated and respected within and beyond the therapy room. By acknowledging our fallibility, learning from our mistakes, and embracing cultural consciousness, we pave the way for a more inclusive, compassionate, and understanding society.

Nurturing Cultural Consciousness: Unravelling Ingrained Biases and Promoting Inclusivity in Everyday Life

In today's interconnected world, fostering cultural consciousness is essential to dismantle biases, promote inclusivity, and create a more harmonious society. It requires individuals to engage in self-reflection, challenge their preconceptions, and actively work towards embracing diverse perspectives. This section will explore practical tips and strategies to help individuals challenge ingrained biases and promote cultural consciousness in their everyday lives, fostering a more inclusive and equitable world.

Self-Reflection: Acknowledge and Challenge Implicit Biases

Begin by reflecting on your own biases, both overt and implicit. Recognise that prejudices are deeply ingrained and influenced by societal norms and conditioning. Engage in self-assessment to identify any discriminatory beliefs or stereotypes you may hold. This critical first step allows you to challenge and replace biased thoughts with more inclusive perspectives consciously and consciously challenge and replace biased opinions with more inclusive views.

Education and Exposure: Seek Knowledge and Diverse Perspectives

Expand your understanding of diverse cultures, histories, and experiences. Read books, watch documentaries, and listen to podcasts that explore diverse narratives. Actively seek out cultural events, exhibitions, and performances to immerse yourself in various experiences. Engaging with multiple voices and perspectives broadens your understanding and helps dismantle stereotypes.

Meaningful Interactions: Embrace Diversity and Foster Empathy

Actively engage with individuals from diverse backgrounds. Initiate conversations, listen attentively, and show genuine curiosity and empathy. Practice active listening, seeking to understand rather than judge. By fostering connections and building bridges, you can challenge assumptions and learn from others' experiences, nurturing a more inclusive mindset.

Allyship and Advocacy: Amplify Marginalised Voices

Stand up as an ally and advocate for marginalised communities. Use your privilege and platform to raise awareness, support initiatives, and promote inclusivity. Amplify marginalised voices by sharing their stories, experiences, and perspectives. Actively contribute your time, skills, and resources to organisations and movements striving for equality and social justice.

Continuous Growth: Embrace Discomfort and Unlearn Biases

Cultivate a mindset of continuous growth by embracing discomfort and being open to unlearning biases. Engage in ongoing self-reflection, seeking feedback from others, and actively challenging your assumptions and prejudices. Embrace diverse viewpoints, even when they question your existing beliefs. This commitment to growth fuels personal transformation and helps break free from ingrained biases.

Cultivate Cultural Intelligence: Embrace Diversity as a Strength

Cultural intelligence involves understanding, appreciating, and adapting to diverse cultures. Educate yourself on cultural norms, customs, and practices. Develop cross-cultural communication skills and strive to be respectful and inclusive. Embracing diversity as a strength enhances your cultural consciousness and fosters inclusive environments.

Engage in Social Justice Movements: Create Lasting Change

Take part in social justice movements and initiatives aimed at dismantling systemic biases. Advocate for policy changes that promote equity and inclusivity. Support organisations are working towards social justice through donations, volunteering, or active participation. You contribute to more significant societal shifts by joining collective efforts and creating lasting change.

Promoting cultural consciousness requires personal growth, self-reflection, and active engagement with diverse perspectives. By acknowledging biases, seeking knowledge, fostering empathy, and advocating for marginalised communities, individuals can challenge ingrained biases and contribute to a more inclusive society. Embrace the tips in this guide and join the collective effort to promote cultural consciousness in your everyday life. Together, we can create a brighter and more inclusive future for all.

Unveiling the Path: Advocating for Culturally Responsive Mental Health Care

Growing up as a Black person, I faced the harsh realities of white superiority, racism, and the lasting impacts of colonialism and neocolonialism on my mental health and that of my community. The erasure of traditional African religions and cultural practices and the imposition of Christianity and Western cultural values further exacerbated our struggles. These experiences shaped my journey to understanding the importance of advocating for our mental health needs and seeking culturally responsive care.

In my younger years, I lacked awareness of how these oppressive systems affected my mental well-being. Only when I decided to pursue therapy did I discover culturally conscious treatment, which connected the dots between my experiences as a Black person and my mental health challenges. This approach taught me to embrace and celebrate my cultural identity, recognising that my heritage could be a source of strength and resilience.

Unfortunately, many Black individuals still lack access to culturally conscious therapy or mental health resources. The persisting disparities in mental health outcomes between Black and white communities highlight the urgent need for systemic change. Our mental health system must acknowledge and respect cultural diversity while addressing the root causes of mental health problems for Black people, including systemic racism, discrimination, and social inequality.

As both a Black person and a culturally conscious therapist, I am committed to playing my part in fostering healing and growth within my community. By acknowledging and celebrating diverse cultural experiences and identities, we can work towards a more just and equitable society. It is essential to dismantling the oppressive systems that have caused immense harm and ensure that everyone, regardless of race, ethnicity, or cultural background, has access to the care needed for their well-being.

The impact of colonialism and racism on the mental health of Black people cannot be understated. The suppression and denigration of traditional African religions and cultural practices during the colonial era severed our connection to our cultural heritage, resulting in a loss of identity and meaning. This dislocation and alienation can contribute to mental health problems like depression and anxiety. The continuous effects of systemic racism and discrimination further exacerbate these challenges.

Moreover, the white saviour narrative perpetuated by neocolonialism, charity, and foreign aid has detrimental effects on the mental health of Black individuals. It reinforces feelings of Black inferiority and dependence on white benevolence, fostering powerlessness and a belief that we cannot help ourselves. Foreign aid often comes with conditions perpetuating poverty and inequality, exacerbating mental health disparities.

To promote mental health and well-being among Black people, we must address the impact of systemic racism, discrimination, and social inequality. Culturally conscious therapy offers a safe and supportive space for individuals to explore the intersection of their cultural identity and mental health, recognising the influence of culture, race, and ethnicity.

Moreover, implementing social and economic policies that address systemic inequalities contributes to better mental health outcomes for Black people and other cultural minorities. By acknowledging and celebrating the diversity of cultural experiences and identities, we can create a society where everyone has equal access to the care needed to thrive.

Addressing these disparities necessitates a comprehensive approach that tackles the root causes of systemic racism and social inequality. It involves implementing policies and programs that address the social determinants of mental health, such as poverty, healthcare access, and discrimination. Additionally, fostering cultural consciousness and inclusivity in mental health care ensures that Black and other cultural minorities receive culturally appropriate care that caters to their unique needs and experiences.

Furthermore, addressing the ongoing effects of colonialism and neocolonialism requires critically examining the underlying systems of power and privilege that perpetuate them. Genuine and equitable partnerships between nations based on mutual respect and understanding are vital. Supporting local initiatives and organisations led by Black people, rather than imposing Western-style solutions, is crucial. We can improve Black people's mental health and well-being by promoting authentic partnerships and addressing the root causes of systemic inequality.

I have experienced the detrimental impact of oppressive systems on mental health. Through my journey, I have discovered the transformative power of culturally conscious therapy and the importance of advocating for mental health needs. I am committed to fostering healing and growth within my community and working towards a mental health system that reflects the diversity of cultural experiences and identities.

Together, we can create a society where everyone has equal access to the care they need to thrive, irrespective of race, ethnicity, or cultural background.

Culturally Responsive Care: Empowering Individuals to Advocate for Their Mental Health

In today's diverse world, it is essential to recognise that mental health needs are not one-size-fits-all. People's experiences, identities, and cultural backgrounds uniquely shape their mental health journey. It is crucial to foster cultural consciousness within the mental health system to provide adequate care. This section explores how individuals can advocate for their mental health needs, seek culturally conscious care, and highlight the transformative power of cultural consciousness.

Recap: Understanding Cultural Consciousness

In Chapter 2, we explored the significance of cultural consciousness in mental health care. Mental health professionals must recognise and respect individuals' diverse backgrounds, identities, and experiences. Cultural consciousness acknowledges the powerful influence of culture on mental health, emphasising the need to tailor care to meet each person's unique needs and preferences.

By embracing cultural consciousness, we can create a safe and inclusive environment where individuals feel seen, heard, and validated. This approach fosters trust and facilitates open communication, enabling others to share their experiences more freely. It also helps break down barriers and challenges that arise from cultural differences, ensuring that mental health care is practical and relevant for all individuals.

In becoming culturally conscious, we must continuously educate ourselves about different cultures, histories, and lived experiences. We must engage in self-reflection to identify and challenge our self-reflection to identify and challenge our biases and misconceptions. Doing so can create a compassionate and empathetic therapeutic space where everyone's unique identity and background are celebrated and respected.

Ultimately, embracing cultural consciousness is not just a professional responsibility but a commitment to understanding and supporting the diverse humanity we serve. As we continue on this path, we contribute to building a more inclusive and equitable society that empowers and uplifts individuals from all walks of life.

Empowering Cultural Consciousness: Self-Advocacy for Culturally Conscious Mental Health Care

1. **Self-Advocacy: Recognising Your Needs and Rights:** The first step in advocating for your mental health needs is recognising and acknowledging them. Reflect on your cultural background, values, beliefs, and the specific challenges or experiences that may impact your well-being. Understanding that you have the right to receive culturally conscious care that respects your identity and meets your unique needs is essential.

2. **Building a Supportive Network:** Seeking support from like-minded individuals who share your cultural background or have had similar experiences can be immensely helpful. Engage in communities, support groups, or online platforms to connect with others who understand and validate your mental health journey. Sharing your experiences and learning from others can empower you to advocate for culturally conscious care.

3. **Educating Yourself and Mental Health Providers:** Knowledge is power. Take the initiative to educate yourself about mental

health and cultural considerations. Learn about the impact of culture on mental health, the potential biases within the mental health system, and the importance of cultural responsiveness. When seeking care, ask potential providers about their experience and training working with diverse populations. Advocate for mental health professionals who prioritise cultural consciousness and are willing to learn and grow in this area.

4. **Assertive Communication: Articulating Your Needs:** Assertive communication is vital when interacting with mental health professionals, the workplace and society. Clearly express your mental health concerns, cultural background, and any specific accommodations or preferences you may have. Please share your story and experiences, helping them understand your unique perspective. Remember that you are the expert on your affairs, and your voice matters.

5. **Collaborative Treatment Planning:** Culturally conscious care is a collaborative process between you and your mental health provider. Actively participate in your treatment planning, discussing your goals, preferences, and cultural considerations. Collaboratively develop strategies that resonate with your cultural background,

incorporate your strengths, and effectively address your mental health concerns.

6. **Seeking Culturally Conscious Providers:**
    Finding mental health providers who prioritise cultural consciousness can be crucial to your well-being. Seek recommendations from trusted sources, such as community organisations, cultural centres, or online directories specialising in culturally conscious care. Take the time to research potential providers, looking for evidence of their commitment to cultural consciousness and inclusivity.

7. **Embracing Cultural Consciousness:**
    Lastly, cultivating cultural consciousness within yourself is a lifelong journey. Reflect on your own biases, assumptions, and preconceptions. Engage in ongoing education and self-reflection to deepen your understanding of diverse cultures, identities, and mental health experiences. Embrace cultural humility, recognising that you can learn from and be influenced by others.

By advocating for their mental health needs and seeking culturally conscious care, individuals can foster positive change within the mental health system. The personal story shared earlier demonstrates cultural consciousness's transformative power and individual advocacy's importance. Remember, your mental health matters; you deserve care that recognises and honours your unique cultural identity. Embrace your voice, educate yourself, and collaborate with culturally conscious providers to ensure your mental well-being is nurtured with empathy, understanding, and cultural consciousness.

Transforming Societal Structures and Norms for Inclusive Mental Well-being: Embracing Cultural Consciousness and its Family of Approaches

In a diverse and interconnected world, creating a society that values and supports the mental well-being of individuals from all racial and cultural backgrounds is crucial. To achieve this, societal structures and norms must undergo transformational changes that embrace cultural consciousness and its approaches, including cultural responsiveness, competency, awareness, intelligence, and sensitivity. This section will explore how these concepts can be applied to create an inclusive society that prioritises mental well-being for all.

Cultural Consciousness: Building Awareness and Recognition

Cultural consciousness serves as the foundation for transforming societal structures and norms. It involves cultivating an understanding and recognition of one's own cultural identity and the cultural identities of others. By fostering cultural consciousness, individuals and communities become more sensitive to the diverse experiences, values, and needs of different racial and cultural backgrounds.

Example: Implementing cultural consciousness education programs to encourage students to explore their cultural heritage and develop an appreciation for other cultures.

Cultural Responsiveness: Addressing Unique Needs and Preferences

Cultural responsiveness goes beyond awareness and actively addresses individuals' unique needs and preferences from diverse backgrounds. It requires adapting practices, policies, and services to be culturally appropriate and respectful. By embracing cultural responsiveness, societal structures and institutions can ensure that mental health support systems are accessible and tailored to the specific cultural contexts of different communities.

Example: Mental health clinics hire diverse staff members and offer culturally sensitive therapeutic approaches that acknowledge and incorporate cultural values and traditions into treatment plans.

Cultural Competency: Enhancing Knowledge and Skills

Cultural competency involves acquiring the knowledge and skills to interact with individuals from diverse cultural backgrounds effectively. It enables professionals and institutions to provide inclusive and equitable support to individuals of all races and cultures. Artistic competency training equips individuals with the tools to navigate cultural differences sensitively and ensures that mental health services are provided without perpetuating cultural biases or stereotypes.

Example: Training mental health practitioners on the specific mental health challenges faced by different racial and cultural communities, along with strategies for culturally appropriate assessment and treatment.

Cultural Awareness: Recognising and Appreciating Diversity

Cultural awareness is an essential aspect of transforming societal structures and norms. It involves recognising and appreciating the existence of diverse cultural groups' values, traditions, and perspectives. By fostering cultural awareness, society can move away from a monolithic understanding of mental well-being and embrace a more pluralistic and inclusive approach.

Example: Hosting community events and gatherings that celebrate the cultural diversity of a neighbourhood, fostering dialogue and understanding among different racial and cultural groups.

Cultural Sensitivity: Respecting and Avoiding Assumptions

Cultural sensitivity is pivotal in transforming societal structures and norms to support mental well-being. It entails being aware and respectful of cultural differences and avoiding assumptions, stereotypes, or judgments based on cultural backgrounds. Culturally sensitive approaches acknowledge the influence of culture on mental health and ensure that support systems consider the unique experiences and needs of diverse racial and cultural communities.

Example: Developing mental health awareness campaigns incorporating culturally diverse narratives and images to resonate with individuals from diverse backgrounds.

Transforming societal structures and norms to create a society that values and supports the mental well-being of individuals from all racial and cultural backgrounds requires an integrated approach rooted in cultural consciousness and its related concepts. By promoting cultural responsiveness, competency, awareness, intelligence, and sensitivity, we can cultivate an inclusive society where mental well-being is prioritised, and everyone has equitable access to culturally appropriate support systems. Embracing these approaches will not only foster individual mental well-being but also contribute to a more just, compassionate, and harmonious society as a whole.

Building a Culture of Mental Well-being: Transforming Societal Structures and Norms

In our quest to create a society that values and supports the mental well-being of individuals from all racial and cultural backgrounds, it is essential to explore tangible steps that can be taken to transform societal structures and norms. Incorporating cultural consciousness, responsiveness, competency, awareness, intelligence, and sensitivity into every aspect of our society can lay the foundation for a more inclusive and equitable future. This section will delve into the strategies, facts, statistics, examples, and case studies that illustrate the transformative power of embracing cultural diversity in fostering mental well-being.

- **Education and Awareness:** One of the fundamental pillars of change lies in education and awareness. Integrating culturally diverse perspectives into educational curricula can cultivate empathy, understanding, and appreciation for diverse cultures. Research has shown that inclusive educational environments positively impact mental well-being, reducing feelings of isolation and enhancing self-esteem among individuals from communities. For example, a study by the American Psychological Association found that students who received multicultural education reported higher well-being and reduced stress levels.

- **Policy Reform:** Policy reform is essential to create a society that genuinely supports the mental well-being of all individuals. Addressing the unique mental health needs and challenges faced by individuals from diverse racial and cultural backgrounds requires targeted initiatives. By allocating resources to underserved communities and promoting diversity in mental health professions, we can bridge the existing gaps in access to care. A prime example of policy reform is the Mental Health Parity and Addiction Equity Act in the United States, which ensures that mental health services are covered at the same level as physical health services, removing a significant barrier to care.

- **Representation and Inclusion:** Representation shapes societal norms and structures. Increasing diversity and inclusion in positions of power and decision-making is essential for creating policies that address the mental health needs of all individuals.

  A study published in the International Journal of Health Services found that ethnic minority patients were more likely to access mental health services when treated by providers of the same ethnic background. This highlights the importance of diversifying the mental health workforce and ensuring culturally conscious care.

- **Culturally Conscious Services:** Access to culturally conscious mental health services is crucial for promoting mental well-being. Recognising and addressing the unique experiences, challenges, and barriers faced by individuals from different racial and cultural backgrounds is essential in providing adequate care. Culturally conscious therapies, such as narrative therapy or Afrocentric approaches, have shown promising results in addressing mental health concerns specific to particular communities.

For instance, a case study conducted in a Hispanic neighbourhood in California showed that incorporating culturally responsive therapy significantly improved treatment outcomes for individuals struggling with depression and anxiety.

- **Community Engagement and Empowerment:** Community engagement is a powerful catalyst for transforming societal structures. We can identify and address specific mental health needs by collaborating with community organisations, leaders, and individuals from diverse backgrounds. The success of community-driven initiatives can be seen in various contexts.

For example, the Well London program in the UK engaged local communities in designing and implementing mental health interventions, resulting in improved mental well-being and increased community cohesion.

- **Addressing Social Determinants of Mental Health:** Creating a society that values and supports mental well-being requires addressing the underlying social determinants that impact mental health outcomes. Systemic racism, socioeconomic disparities, and access to quality healthcare, affordable housing, and education significantly influence mental well-being.

Australia's Mental Health Matters initiative exemplifies a comprehensive approach to addressing these determinants. This program focuses on promoting mental health literacy, addressing stigma, and addressing the social factors contributing to mental health inequities.

Transforming societal structures and norms to create a society that values and supports the mental well-being of individuals from all racial and cultural backgrounds is an ongoing journey. By integrating cultural consciousness, responsiveness, competency, awareness, intelligence, and sensitivity into the fabric of our society, we can foster a sense of belonging and empower individuals to seek help and support.

We can build a culture where mental well-being knows no boundaries through education, policy reform, representation, culturally conscious services, community engagement, and addressing social determinants. The path to change requires collective efforts, but the benefits are immeasurable. By embracing diversity, fostering cultural understanding, and prioritising mental well-being for all, we create a society that thrives on inclusivity, compassion, and equity.

Let us embark on this transformative journey together and build a future where everyone, regardless of their racial or cultural background, can experience the support, validation, and care we deserve for our mental well-being.

A Brighter Future: A Journey Towards Mental Freedom

As we conclude this book on transforming societal structures and norms to prioritise the mental well-being of individuals from all racial and cultural backgrounds, it is essential to reflect on the significance of our collective efforts. Throughout this journey, we have explored the power of cultural consciousness, responsiveness, competency, awareness, intelligence, and sensitivity in dismantling barriers and promoting mental freedom. Now, let us envision a brighter future that may not manifest in our lifetimes but inspires us to use our voices, borne from experiences of marginalisation, discrimination, and allyship, to rally for emancipation from mental slavery into mental freedom.

A World Transformed:

In the future, I envision, mental well-being is not a luxury but a fundamental human right. It is a world where every individual feels seen, heard, and valued for their unique experiences and cultural identities. The societal structures and norms that once perpetuated stigmas and inequalities are replaced with inclusivity, empathy, and understanding. Mental health is destigmatised and openly discussed, fostering a culture of compassion and support.

Education as Empowerment:

In this future, education systems are not only a tool for knowledge and oppression but also a tool for knowledge and oppression and a vehicle for empowerment. Curricula embrace diversity, acknowledging the historical contributions and resilience of marginalised communities. Children grow up with a deep understanding and appreciation for diverse cultures, fostering empathy and breaking down the walls of ignorance and prejudice. Mental health education is prioritised, equipping individuals with the necessary skills to navigate their emotional well-being and support others.

Policies of Equality:

The future we strive for will be shaped by policies that champion equality and justice. Governments and institutions are committed to eradicating systemic barriers disproportionately affecting marginalised individuals. Mental health services are accessible and affordable, with resources distributed equitably to address the specific needs of diverse communities. Policies promote diversity and inclusion in the mental health workforce, ensuring culturally conscious care for all.

Representation as Empathy:

In this future, representation is not a token gesture but a powerful force for empathy and understanding. Voices of marginalised individuals are amplified, and positions of influence reflect the rich tapestry of humanity. Decision-makers understand the nuances and complexities of diverse experiences, shaping policies that foster mental well-being for all. Through representation, we validate the struggles and triumphs of individuals from different racial and cultural backgrounds, fostering a sense of belonging and collective progress.

Community, Support, and Healing:

Communities are at the heart of this brighter future. They are spaces of support where individuals come together to share their journeys, offer solace, and heal collectively. Community organisations thrive, providing culturally responsive and holistic support systems that celebrate diversity and prioritise mental well-being. Together, communities challenge the societal narratives that perpetuate discrimination and embrace the power of unity in fostering mental freedom.

A Call to Action:

As we conclude this book, I am honoured to stand alongside my fellow warriors against marginalisation and discrimination. Each of us carries a unique story, a voice that can spark change. Let us use our experiences to fuel our advocacy for mental freedom, knowing that our efforts ripple through time, shaping a future where the mental well-being of all individuals is cherished and protected.

I am inspired by the late Nelson Mandela, Martin Luther King, Malcolm X, and Gandhi. Inspired by their unwavering commitment to justice, equality, and liberation, I carry their spirit within me as I navigate the path ahead. Like Mandela, I strive to break down the walls of mental oppression, promoting healing and reconciliation. Like King, I dream of a society where individuals are judged not by the colour of their skin or cultural background but by the content of their character. Like Malcolm X, I seek to empower individuals to embrace their identity, unapologetically advocating for their mental well-being. Like Gandhi, I believe in the transformative power of nonviolent resistance, using my voice to peacefully challenge the status quo and dismantle the barriers that hinder mental freedom.

Though we may not witness the full realisation of this vision in our lifetimes, our commitment to the cause ensures that the torch is passed on. Let us empower the next generation to carry forward the fight, armed with knowledge, resilience, and the unwavering belief in the power of unity and understanding. Together, we can pave the way to a brighter future, where mental freedom is a birthright and individuals from all racial and cultural backgrounds thrive in a society that uplifts and supports their well-being.

Closing Words:

In closing, I invite you to embrace the power within you, the power of your voice, and your experiences. By standing up for mental freedom and advocating for the well-being of all individuals, we honour the legacies of those who came before us. Let us be the change we wish to see in the world, forging a path towards a brighter future where mental freedom knows no boundaries. May our collective efforts resonate through the generations, bringing us closer to the day when all individuals, regardless of their racial or cultural background, experience the profound liberation of true mental well-being.

Summary:

This powerful and enlightening book explores the profound impact of cultural consciousness in transforming societal structures, norms, mental health practices, workplaces, and individual lives. By delving into cultural responsiveness, competency, awareness, intelligence, sensitivity, and empathy, we uncover the key ingredients needed to create a society that values and supports the mental well-being of individuals from all racial and cultural backgrounds.

Throughout the book, we discover that cultural consciousness plays a pivotal role in shaping mental health practices. By recognising the influence of culture on mental well-being, professionals can develop culturally conscious approaches that tailor interventions, incorporate diverse perspectives, and address the disparities in access to care. This leads to improved outcomes and a more equitable mental health system.

We also explore the importance of cultivating culturally conscious workplaces. By fostering an inclusive environment that respects and celebrates diverse cultural backgrounds, organisations can promote mental health awareness, provide support mechanisms, and address workplace stressors that may disproportionately affect individuals from different racial and cultural backgrounds. Creating inclusive workplaces benefits employees' mental well-being and enhances productivity, collaboration, and overall organisational success.

However, transforming societal structures requires a more profound commitment to challenging deeply rooted biases, stereotypes, and systemic inequalities. By promoting cultural consciousness and inclusivity, we can actively dismantle barriers that hinder the mental well-being of individuals from marginalised communities. This involves confronting racism, discrimination, and social inequities contributing to mental health disparities. We can pave the way for a more just and equitable society through collective efforts and advocacy.

At the individual level, cultural consciousness empowers us to recognise our biases, increase empathy, and actively dismantle oppressive systems. By embracing our role as change agents, we can advocate for our mental health needs, seek culturally responsive care, and support others in their journey toward mental well-being. Each individual's journey contributes to a more significant movement, inspiring others and creating a ripple effect of positive change.

By embracing cultural consciousness, promoting inclusivity in mental health practices, workplaces, and society, and empowering individuals, we can collectively pave the way toward a future where mental well-being is valued, supported, and accessible to all. This future is within our grasp, and with dedication, collaboration, and unwavering commitment, we can build a society that genuinely celebrates and nurtures the mental health of every individual, regardless of their racial or cultural background.

Chapter 6 Key Points:

Mental Health Practices: Culturally conscious approaches in mental health practices emphasise recognising and integrating cultural factors that influence individuals' mental well-being. This includes tailoring therapeutic interventions, incorporating diverse perspectives, and addressing cultural disparities in access to care.

Workplaces: Creating culturally conscious workplaces involves fostering an inclusive environment that respects and celebrates diverse cultural backgrounds. This includes promoting mental health awareness, providing support mechanisms, and addressing workplace stressors that may disproportionately affect individuals from different racial and cultural backgrounds.

Society: Transforming societal structures and norms necessitates challenging deeply rooted biases, stereotypes, and systemic inequalities. By promoting cultural consciousness and inclusivity, society can actively dismantle barriers that hinder the mental well-being of individuals from marginalised communities.

Individuals: Cultivating cultural consciousness on an individual level enables people to recognise their own biases, increase empathy, and actively engage in dismantling oppressive systems. It empowers individuals to advocate for their mental health needs, seek culturally responsive care, and support others in their journey toward mental well-being.

Key Takeaways:

Cultural consciousness is a catalyst:

- Recognising the influence of culture on mental well-being is essential for creating effective mental health practices.
- Fostering inclusive workplaces.
- Promoting a society that values and supports diverse individuals.

Inclusivity in mental health practices:

- Embracing culturally responsive approaches in mental health practices ensures that care is tailored to individuals' unique needs and experiences, leading to better outcomes and reduced disparities.

Culturally conscious workplaces:

- Building inclusive workplaces requires acknowledging and celebrating diversity.
- Promoting mental health awareness.
- Providing support mechanisms that recognise the impact of culture on employees' well-being.

Challenging societal norms:

- Transforming societal structures involves actively challenging biases, stereotypes, and systemic inequalities perpetuating mental health disparities among individuals from different racial and cultural backgrounds.

Empowered individuals:

- Cultivating cultural consciousness empowers individuals to advocate for their mental health needs, seek culturally conscious care, and actively contribute to dismantling oppressive systems in pursuit of mental freedom.

Collaborative efforts:

- Creating a society that values and supports mental well-being for all necessitates collaboration among mental health professionals, community organisations, workplaces, and individuals from diverse backgrounds.

A future of mental well-being:

- By embracing cultural consciousness, promoting inclusivity, and prioritising mental health at all levels, we can envision a future where mental well-being is valued, supported, and accessible to individuals from all racial and cultural backgrounds.

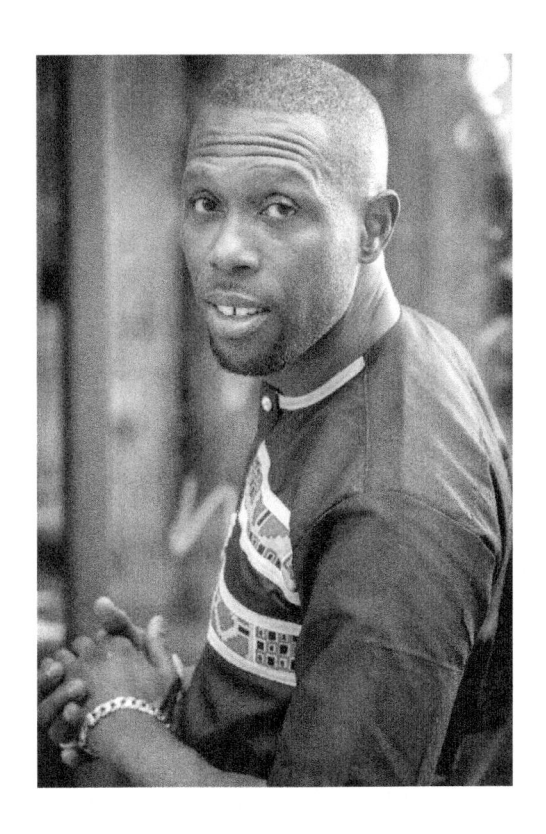

About the Author

Get ready to be inspired by the visionary behind the groundbreaking book, "White Talking Therapy Can't Think in Black - A Guide to Healing from Systemic Racism." Jarell Bempong, a dynamic catalyst for change, personifies the spirit of transformation, ceaselessly advocating for healing, equity, and cultural inclusion within the mental health landscape.

Jarell's journey is rooted in firsthand experiences that have shaped his unwavering commitment to confront and dismantle the oppressive systems perpetuating systemic racism and discrimination. He draws upon extensive expertise as a psychotherapist, counsellor, transformational coach, speaker, and trainer to ignite a global change movement.

Growing up, Jarell intimately witnessed the destructive impact of white supremacy and privilege, an experience that lit the fire of his passion for justice. His family dynamics, with a Black Ghanaian Mother, Black Brother, White English stepfather and mixed-race siblings, provided a lens through which he understood the insidious nature of racism. Jarell's Ghanaian heritage further enriched his perspective, allowing him to grasp the lasting consequences of slavery and colonialism on African societies. Armed with this comprehensive understanding, Jarell fearlessly challenges harmful narratives and amplifies the voices of marginalised communities.

His expertise extends far beyond the boundaries of traditional therapy. He recognises that mental well-being is intricately intertwined with the broader social determinants that shape our lives. By delving into the depths of systemic racism, discrimination, and social inequality, Jarell illuminates the root causes of mental health disparities. Through his work, he strives to build bridges between cultural identities, foster inclusivity, and empower individuals to embrace their strengths and cultural resources.

As an advocate for racial inclusion and parity, Jarell understands that change must occur on both individual and systemic levels. His deep commitment to cultural consciousness, allyship and antiracism informs his approach to therapy, training, and public speaking engagements. Jarell's international reach as a speaker and trainer allows him to engage diverse audiences in robust discussions about mental health, diversity, equality, inclusion, and intersectionality. He is a catalyst for transformative conversations, challenging societal norms, and redefining the parameters of creating an inclusive and equitable world.

Jarell Bempong's journey embodies resilience, empathy, and expertise. His fusion of academic knowledge with lived experiences propels him to the forefront of the mental health reform movement. By sharing his insights, personal anecdotes, and practical strategies, Jarell empowers mental health professionals, the workforce, and individuals to dismantle the oppressive structures that impede progress.

"White Talking Therapy Can't Think in Black - A Guide to Healing from Systemic Racism" is a powerful call to action, urging readers to challenge the status quo, recognise their biases, and actively contribute to a more just and equitable society. Jarell's unwavering dedication to healing, equity, and cultural inclusion offers a beacon of hope and inspiration to all those seeking to navigate the complex intersection of mental health, systemic racism, and societal change.

Prepare to embark on a transformative journey guided by Jarell Bempong's expert knowledge, compassionate insight, and unyielding commitment to decolonising mental health. Together, we can forge a path towards healing, justice, and a future where everyone's well-being is valued and supported, regardless of their racial or cultural background.

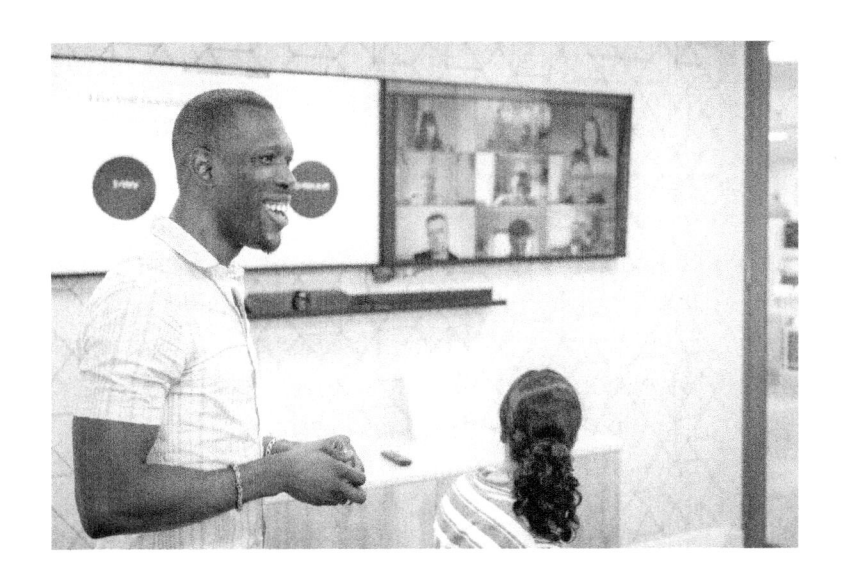

Services by Jarell Bempong: Expanding the Journey

Jall Bempong, a specialist culturally conscious psychotherapist, counsellor, transformational coach, speaker, and trainer, extends his passion for promoting mental health equity and inclusivity through a diverse range of offerings beyond his groundbreaking book, "White Talking Therapy Can't Think in Black - A Guide to Healing from Systemic Racism."

- **Engaging Keynotes and Workshops:** Unleash the power of Jarell's dynamic speaking engagements and workshops. With his captivating presence and interactive approach,

Jarell creates a space for thought-provoking discussions on mental health, diversity, equality, and inclusion. Prepare to be inspired and equipped with practical tools for driving meaningful change.

- **Culturally Conscious Therapy:** Experience the transformative impact of Jarell's culturally conscious therapy at www.bempongtalkingtherapy.com. Recognising the unique needs of individuals from diverse backgrounds, Jarell provides an empathetic and inclusive therapeutic environment. Through his guidance, you can navigate your mental health challenges and contribute to a more inclusive and just society.
- **Consulting and Coaching Services:** Organizations committed to fostering diversity, equality, and inclusion can benefit from Jarell's comprehensive consulting and coaching services. With his expertise, Jarell guides organisations in developing strategies, policies, and frameworks that create a culturally responsive and equitable environment. Take a proactive step towards positive change and growth.
- **Empowering Webinars and Online Courses:** Embark on a transformative learning journey through Jarell's engaging webinars and online courses. Dive deep into key topics and gain the knowledge and skills to drive meaningful change at your own pace. Unlock your potential and become an agent of change in your personal and professional life.

- **Promoting Racial Inclusion:** Join Jarell in his unwavering commitment to racial inclusion and parity. Through his work, he strives to enhance the quality of life for individuals from diverse ethnic backgrounds. Break free from the constraints of racial and cultural biases, fostering optimal mental well-being, career growth, and overall development.

Jarell Bempong's offerings expand the journey beyond the pages of his book, inviting you to engage, learn, and actively contribute to a more inclusive world. Explore these empowering resources and services to ignite transformative conversations and create lasting change.

Contact Jarell Bempong today to discover how his services can support your organisation or to inquire about captivating keynotes and workshops:

Email: info@bempongtalkingtherapy.com

Phone: 020 3059 9459

Website: www.bempongtalkingtherapy.com

Linkedin: linkedin.com/in/jarellbempong/

Instagram: instagram.com/bempongtalkingtherapy/

Printed in Great Britain
by Amazon